To my dear wife Kimberley and our children, Thomas and Ella, and also to my parents.
David C. Howlett

To my wife Vanessa and our children, Thomas, Benjamin, Harriet and Emily.
Michael P. Saunders

Cases in
Surgical Radiology

EDITED BY

David C. Howlett MRCP FRCR
Michael P. Saunders BSc MS FRCS

Eastbourne District General Hospital
Kings Drive
Eastbourne
BN21 2UD

FOREWORD BY

Martin H. Jourdan

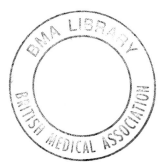

**Blackwell
Science**

© 2001 by
Blackwell Science Ltd
Editorial Offices:
Osney Mead, Oxford OX2 0EL
25 John Street, London WC1N 2BS
23 Ainslie Place, Edinburgh EH3 6AJ
350 Main Street, Malden
   MA 02148-5018, USA
54 University Street, Carlton
   Victoria 3053, Australia
10, rue Casimir Delavigne
   75006 Paris, France

Other Editorial Offices:
Blackwell Wissenschafts-Verlag GmbH
Kurfürstendamm 57
10707 Berlin, Germany

Blackwell Science KK
MG Kodenmacho Building
7–10 Kodenmacho Nihombashi
Chuo-ku, Tokyo 104, Japan

Iowa State University Press
A Blackwell Science Company
2121 S. State Avenue
Ames, Iowa 50014-8300, USA

First published 2001

Set by Graphicraft Limited, Hong Kong
Printed and bound in Great Britain by
MPG Books Ltd., Bodmin, Cornwall

DISTRIBUTORS
Marston Book Services Ltd
PO Box 269
Abingdon, Oxon OX14 4YN
(*Orders*: Tel: 01235 465500
            Fax: 01235 465555)

The Americas
Blackwell Publishing
c/o AIDC
PO Box 20
50 Winter Sport Lane
Williston, VT 05495-0020
(*Orders*: Tel: 800 216 2522
            Fax: 802 864 7626)

Australia
Blackwell Science Pty Ltd
54 University Street
Carlton, Victoria 3053
(*Orders*: Tel: 3 9347 0300
            Fax: 3 9347 5001)

A catalogue record for this title
is available from the British Library

ISBN 0-632-05822-6

Library of Congress
Cataloging-in-Publication Data

Cases in surgical radiology/
edited by David C. Howlett and
Michael P. Saunders; with foreword by
Desmond H. Birkett.
     p. ;   cm.
Includes bibliographical references and
index.
ISBN 0-632-05822-6 (pbk.)
1. Interventional radiology—Case
studies—Problems, exercises, etc.
2. Radiography, Medical—Case studies—
Problems, etc.
3. Diagnostic imaging—Case studies—
Problems, exercises, etc.
I. Howlett, David C.   II. Saunders,
Michael P.
[DNLM: 1. Diagnostic imaging—
methods—Problems and exercises.
2. Diagnosis, differential—problems
and exercise.
WN 18.2 C338 2001]
RD33.55 .C374   2001
617'.0754'076—dc21   2001025163

For further information on
Blackwell Science, visit our website:
www.blackwell-science.com

CONTENTS

LIST OF CONTRIBUTORS

Hugh J. Anderson FRCR
Consultant Radiologist
Eastbourne District General Hospital
Kings Drive
Eastbourne

Stephen G. Ho MD FRCPC
Department of Radiology
Vancouver General Hospital
British Columbia

David C. Howlett MRCP FRCR
Consultant Radiologist
Eastbourne District General Hospital
Kings Drive
Eastbourne

David V. Hughes MRCP FRCR
Consultant Radiologist
Department of Radiology
Eastbourne District General Hospital
Kings Drive
Eastbourne

Nigel D.P. Marchbank MRCP FRCR
Consultant Radiologist
Department of Radiology
Eastbourne District General Hospital
Kings Drive
Eastbourne

Peter L. Munk MD CM FRCPC
Professor of MusculoSkeletal Radiology
Vancouver General Hospital
British Columbia

Sheila C. Rankin FRCR
Consultant Radiologist
Department of Radiology
Guy's & St Thomas' Hospitals
St Thomas' Street
London

Elizabeth Ruffell FRCP FRCR
Consultant Radiologist
Department of Radiology
Eastbourne District General Hospital
Kings Drive
Eastbourne

David F. Sallomi DMRD FRCR
Consultant Radiologist
Department of Radiology
Eastbourne District General Hospital
Kings Drive
Eastbourne

Michael P. Saunders BSc MS FRCS
Consultant Surgeon
Eastbourne District General Hospital
Kings Drive
Eastbourne

FOREWORD

The breathtaking advances in all aspects of radiological investigations in the last few years have meant that the clinician often has a very precise idea of the anatomy and physiology of the patient's problem on which to base management. Surgery can be tailored and planned in advance, and just as importantly those patients who will not benefit can be spared unnecessary exploratory procedures.

This book produced from the experience of Eastbourne, British Columbia, Guy's and St. Thomas' Hospitals fills a much needed niche to correlate the radiological appearances with the diagnosis and subsequent clinical management. The eight chapters, each put together by a different specialist, cover a wide field including gastroenterology, urology, orthopaedics and neurology, and a number of radiological modalities. In each chapter a number of cases are presented in the format of a question on one page, followed by an answer and plan for management on the subsequent page. Each is provided with one pertinent reference for further reading. The editors have managed to keep the text crisp and to the point. The illustrations are good quality which is a must for a production of this kind. One somehow feels that this is just the beginning and there is much scope for further *Cases in Surgical Radiology* in the future.

This book will appeal to all surgeons and radiologists and will be particularly valuable to those preparing for higher examinations such as the MRCS and FRCS in the UK and equivalent examinations elsewhere. Indeed I suspect that medical students will find this an enjoyable and informative exercise in self-assessment.

Martin Jourdan BSc PhD MS FRCS
Consultant Surgeon and Reader in Surgery
Guy's and St Thomas' Hospitals, London

PREFACE

The rapid technological advances occurring in radiology provide a tempting route by which a clinician can gain rapid diagnosis of the patient's condition. However, misdirected investigations may prove inconvenient, cause delay or may indeed be detrimental to patient care. There remains no substitute for a thorough history and careful examination. Radiology can often provide an understanding of the clinical symptoms and signs elicited.

Communicating the key clinical features of a patient's condition is a thought-requiring and necessary skill, which comes to the forefront when details need to be compressed within the limited space of a radiology request form! This necessity forms the theme of *Cases in Surgical Radiology*. Throughout the varied chapters, each generously contributed by colleagues, key clinical features are presented alongside an initial radiological study. Interpretation of the image is provided together with guidance towards the next most appropriate radiological study.

Our aim is to challenge knowledge in surgical radiology. We trust you will find the cases as educative and rewarding as we have during their compilation.

ACKNOWLEDGEMENTS

The authors wish to thank Mrs Helen Perry and Miss Louise Pellett for preparation of the manuscript and Nick Taylor for preparation of the photographs.

CHAPTER 1

Hugh J. Anderson

CASE 1

A 47-year-old man presents with non-specific abdominal discomfort and altered bowel habit.

What abnormality is demonstrated on the supine abdominal radiograph (Fig. 1.1)?
What is the diagnosis and how may this be confirmed radiologically?
What are the important differential diagnoses?

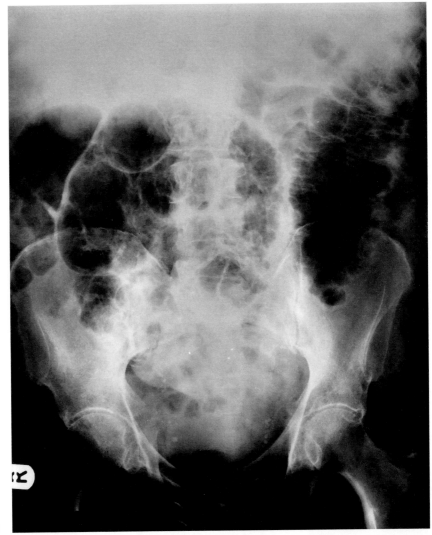

Fig. 1.1

The supine abdominal radiograph (Fig. 1.1) shows multiple air-filled spaces within the wall of the colon. These features are consistent with the diagnosis of pneumatosis cystoides intestinalis. The barium enema radiograph (Fig. 1.2) illustrates this condition well. Multiple radiolucent defects within the bowel wall are present in the region of the left hemicolon (open arrows). These changes extend outside the column of barium. There is coincidental mild sigmoid diverticular disease.

Pneumatosis cystoides intestinalis

• Benign condition characterized by air-filled cysts (up to 3 cm in diameter) within the submucosal or subserosal surfaces of the colon.
• Perforation of subserosal cysts may result in asymptomatic pneumoperitoneum.
• Aetiology remains obscure. Favoured theories include gas-producing organisms, excessive intraluminal fermentation and dissociation of gas under high pressure from the lumen into the bowel wall.
• Male predominance, usually between the ages of 30 and 50 years.

• Association with peptic ulceration and pyloric stenosis, intestinal bypass surgery for morbid obesity and chronic lung disease.
• Hyperbaric oxygen therapy has been used successfully for symptomatic patients.

It is clearly of utmost importance to distinguish the air-filled cysts of pneumatosis cystoides intestinalis from intramural gas. This latter condition usually presents as a linear gas pattern and may be associated with more serious pathologies, notably bowel infarction.

The abdominal radiograph features of pneumatosis cystoides intestinalis may be confused with:
• multiple colonic polyps in familial adenomatous polyposis;
• gas within diverticula;
• faecal material within the colonic lumen.
Distinction between these conditions is achieved by barium enema or CT imaging.

Further reading

Thomas, B. (1993) The colon. In: *A Textbook of Radiology and Imaging* (ed. D. Sutton), 5th edn, p. 872. Churchill Livingstone Publications, Edinburgh.

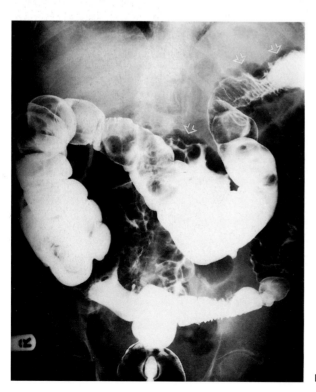

Fig. 1.2

CASE 2

The clinical condition of a young patient with a 2-week history of profuse diarrhoea, pyrexia and abdominal pain worsens with the advent of signs of peritonitis.

What abnormalities are evident on the supine abdominal radiograph (Fig. 1.3)?

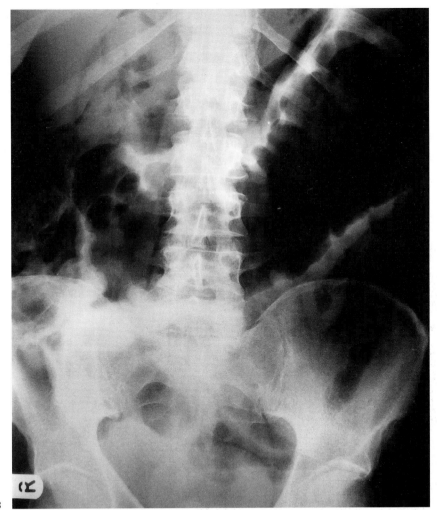

Fig. 1.3

The reproduced abdominal radiograph (Fig. 1.4) illustrates marked dilatation of the transverse colon (white arrows) with gross oedema of the colonic wall. These features are consistent with toxic megacolon. Additionally there are widespread intramural linear gas patterns (small white arrows) as well as free intraperitoneal gas (well seen in the right upper quadrant—open arrow). The features are those of a severe colitis with large bowel perforation.

Differential diagnosis of toxic megacolon

- Ulcerative colitis.
- Crohn's disease.
- Infective colitis (commonly salmonella and amoebic).
- Pseudomembranous colitis.
- Ischaemic colitis.

In this case the diagnosis is salmonella colitis. The infective organism is usually *Salmonella typhi* or *paratyphi* and this may be isolated in stool or blood culture. Normally it is a self-limiting condition and this patient presented with the classic prodromal symptoms of pyrexia, malaise, arthralgia and, later, non-specific abdominal disturbance. Colonic involvement typically affects the descending and sigmoid colon with sparing of the rectum. Pathological changes range from diffuse superficial ulceration to severe pancolitis with deep 'collar-stud' ulceration, mucosal oedema and intramural gas. Colonic perforation is unusual.

Further reading

Glick, S.N. (1994) Other inflammatory conditions of the colon. In *Textbook of Gastrointestinal Radiology* (eds R.M. Gore & M.S. Levine), pp. 993–1008. W.B. Saunders Co., Philadelphia.

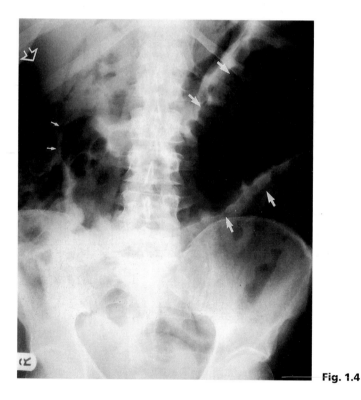

Fig. 1.4

CASE 3

A middle-aged man with long-standing controlled hypertension presented with right iliac fossa discomfort and a palpable pulsatile mass in this region.

What examination is illustrated (Fig. 1.5) and what does it demonstrate?
What would be your first-line imaging modality?
How may the condition be managed?

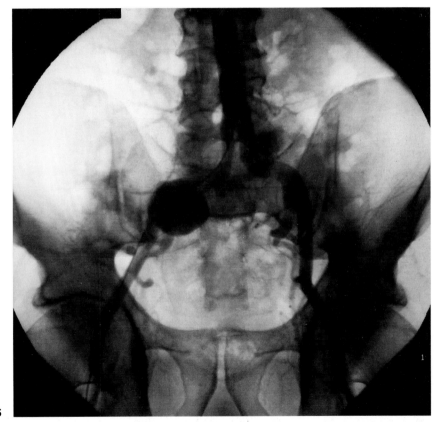

Fig. 1.5

The radiograph (Fig. 1.5) is taken from a digital subtraction angiography (DSA) series. Angiography has been performed via a right femoral approach and demonstrates an aneurysm of the right common iliac artery.

Abdominal/pelvic ultrasound scan is the most appropriate first-line imaging test. This was performed and the diagnosis of an aneurysm was confirmed with the aid of colour Doppler. This was complemented by CT angiography; however, it was not possible to determine whether the aneurysm arose from the right common or internal iliac artery. Angiography (Fig. 1.5) successfully resolved this. MR angiography may also provide similar information.

The options for treatment include surgery and stent grafting. Conventional surgery for this condition has a mortality rate of about 10% in the absence of any significant co-morbidity. The 4-year primary patency rate for stent grafts, at this site, approaches 95%. Stent grafting was chosen and a completion angiogram (Fig. 1.6) confirms exclusion of the aneurysm with the stent *in situ* (arrows).

Potential complications of iliac stent grafts

- Immediate/periprocedural: distal emboli, graft thrombosis, puncture site haemorrhage.
- Long term: 'endo-leak', graft thrombosis.

Further reading

Sanchez, L., Patel, A., Ohki, T. *et al.* (1999) Mid-term experience with the endovascular treatment of isolated iliac aneurysms. *Journal of Vascular Surgery* **30**, 907–913.

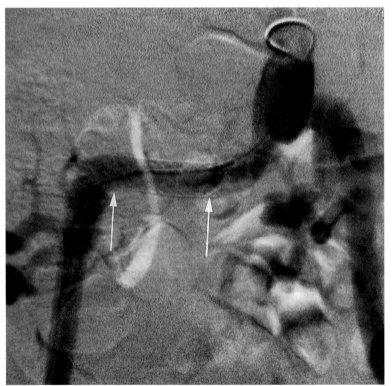

Fig. 1.6

CASE 4

A middle-aged female patient was admitted with a history of severe pain in the right leg for 2 hours. This had lessened, but still required opiate analgesia for pain relief. The patient was found to be in atrial fibrillation. Examination revealed an ischaemic right leg with absent femoral pulse.

What examination is shown (Fig. 1.7) and what abnormality is present?
What alternative imaging techniques could be employed?
What are the management options?

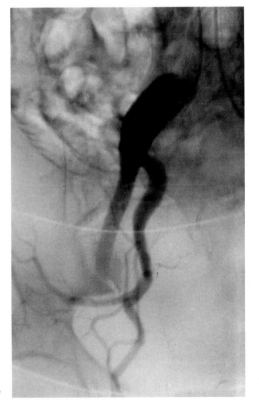

Fig. 1.7

A digital subtraction angiogram (DSA—Fig. 1.7) has been undertaken from a left femoral approach using a 'hook-over' technique across the aortic bifurcation, and this demonstrates an embolic occlusion of the right common femoral artery and its branches.

Alternative imaging techniques include colour Doppler ultrasound and CT/MR angiography. Ultrasound may be helpful in determining both the level of the occlusion and its extent. It is, however, time consuming and requires considerable technical expertise. In common with both CT and MR angiography it is non-invasive and safe. Where management of the patient is likely to involve radiological or surgical intervention, DSA will provide the most detailed information immediately prior to therapeutic intervention.

This clinical situation can be managed either surgically or radiologically depending on the clinical setting and local expertise. This case was managed successfully by low-dose intra-arterial thrombolysis using recombinant tissue plasminogen activator (r-TPA). A postprocedure angiographic image (Fig. 1.8) demonstrates patent common and superficial femoral arteries with some free proximal intraluminal thrombus (arrows). Echocardiography was also performed and confirmed the presence of left atrial thrombus—the embolic source, secondary to the patient's arrhythmia—and oral anticoagulation therapy was also commenced.

Complications of intra-arterial thrombolysis

• Haemorrhage (local, gastrointestinal, intracranial).
• Distal embolization of thrombus.
• Vessel dissection/perforation.
• Pericatheter thrombosis.

Further reading

Belli, A. & Buckenhom, T. (1996) Vascular intervention. In: *Interventional Radiology, a Practical Guide* (eds A. Watkinson & A. Adam), pp. 130–138. Radcliffe Medical Press, New York.

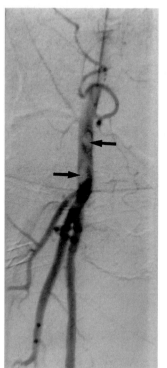

Fig. 1.8

CASE 5

A 17-year-old male with a vague history of odynophagia refused endoscopy. An upper gastrointestinal barium study was performed.

What abnormalities are demonstrated on the images from a barium swallow (Figs 1.9 & 1.10)?
What is the differential diagnosis?
How could the diagnosis be confirmed?

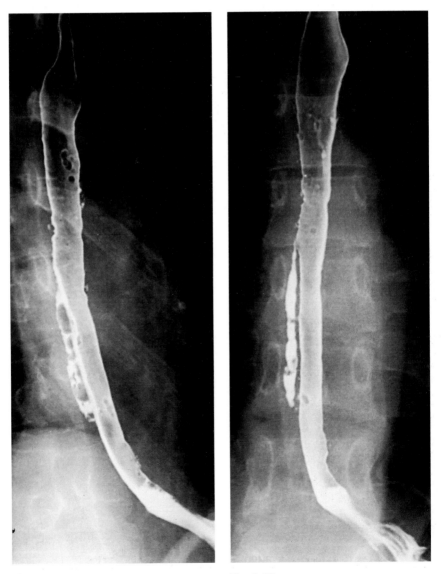

Fig. 1.9   **Fig. 1.10**

The reproduced images from the barium swallow study (Figs 1.11 & 1.12) show appearances of a 'double-barrelled oesophagus'. There are small aphthous-type ulcers (Fig. 1.11, small arrows) highlighted by the effect of small collections of barium within circular or linear superficial ulcers, surrounded by a correspondingly shaped darker area of oedema. Barium is also filling an intramural tract (Fig. 1.12, open arrows) caused by deeper ulceration and the development of an intramural track. These features result from Crohn's disease.

Causes of aphthous/superficial oesophageal ulceration

- Crohn's disease.

- Herpes, cytomegalovirus and other infective oesophagitides.
- Chemical and reflux oesophagitis.
- Drug induced.

Differential diagnosis of intramural tracks

- Crohn's disease.
- Post instrumentation.
- Candidiasis.
- Tuberculosis.

Further reading

Laufer, I. (1989) Other esophagatides. In: *Radiology of the Esophagus* (ed. M.S. Levine), pp. 91–112. W.B. Saunders Co., Philadelphia.

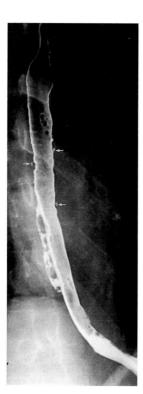

Fig. 1.11

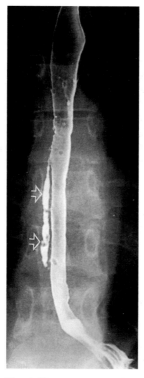

Fig. 1.12

CHAPTER 1

CASE 6

An 83-year-old female diagnosed 3 months previously with inoperable carcinoma of the mid-oesophagus had had palliative treatment involving insertion of a covered self-expanding metallic stent (SEMS). This had afforded good relief of her dysphagia until she re-presented with respiratory difficulties provoked by eating and drinking. A water-soluble contrast swallow examination was undertaken.

Given the above history, what important possible diagnoses should the radiologist be forewarned of and why?
What does this lateral contrast swallow radiograph (Fig. 1.13) show?

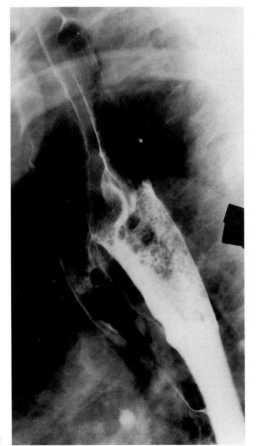

Fig. 1.13

The clinical history raises the possibility of a tracheo-oesophageal fistula or stent occlusion with secondary aspiration. Although barium is relatively inert in the bronchial tree it requires considerable physiotherapy to encourage expectoration. Gastrografin should be avoided in this situation as it is extremely irritant to the lungs and may result in oedema and bronchospasm. The preferred contrast medium is a non-ionic water-soluble product.

The reproduced lateral view (Fig. 1.14) of the contrast swallow demonstrates a tracheo-oesophageal fistula related to the proximal end of the stent (long arrow) with contrast seen within the trachea (small arrows). Reflux with aspiration is not thought to be the cause in this case since contrast is not seen above the level of the stent.

Complications of oesophageal SEMS

- Stent migration.
- Occlusion (bolus, tumour overgrowth/ingrowth).
- Oesophageal rupture.
- Fistula formation (tracheo-oesophageal, aorto-oesophageal).
- Haemorrhage.

In this case the tracheo-oesophageal fistula was successfully treated by deployment of a second covered SEMS within the oesophagus to 'exclude' the fistula. This technique is limited by the level of the fistula because stents deployed high in the oesophagus are not as well tolerated as those placed distally.

Further reading

Mohammed, S. & Moss, J. (1996) Palliation of malignant tracheo-oesophageal fistula using covered metal stents. *Clinical Radiology* **51**, 42–46.

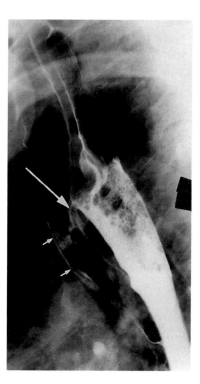

Fig. 1.14

CASE 7

A middle-aged male patient had an emergency intravenous urogram undertaken for left flank pain and pyrexia.

What abnormalities are demonstrated on this radiograph (Fig. 1.15) taken 10 minutes after intravenous contrast administration? (No additional information was present on the initial control abdominal radiograph.) What further imaging may be helpful?

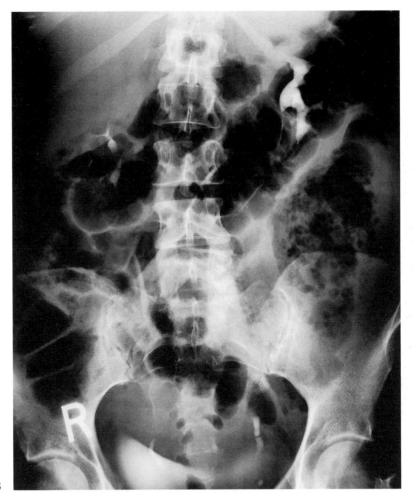

Fig. 1.15

The radiograph (Fig. 1.15) taken during an intravenous urogram demonstrates medial displacement of the left ureter by a left-sided abdominal mass which contains abnormal gas shadows and soft tissue density material. The proximal transverse colon is moderately dilated (7 cm diameter). These appearances are explained by a pericolic abscess complicating left colonic diverticular disease. Extension into the retroperitoneal space has resulted in medial deviation of the left ureter.

Causes of medial deviation of the ureter

- Retroperitoneal fibrosis, tumour, haemorrhage or abscess.
- Enlarged iliac lymph nodes.
- Iliac artery aneurysm.
- Retrocaval ureter (only on the right).

The oblique radiograph (Fig. 1.16) of a barium enema examination taken from a different patient demonstrates a long, irregular, diverticular stricture of the sigmoid colon with tracking of barium outside the bowel lumen into a localized, pericolic abscess (arrows).

Additional imaging will be influenced by the clinical setting. Ultrasound is of limited assistance since bowel gas within a collection interferes with visualization. CT imaging is most useful in assessing the retroperitoneal region and may also be used to aid in the percutaneous insertion of drainage catheters and biopsies. MR imaging may also be helpful, particularly in the evaluation of retroperitoneal tumours.

Further reading

Balthazar, E.J. (2000) Diverticular disease of the colon. In: *Textbook of Gastrointestinal Radiology* (eds R.M. Gore & M.S. Levine), 2nd edn, pp. 915–944. W.B. Saunders Co., Philadelphia.

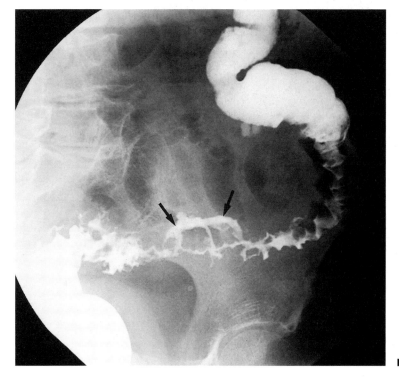

Fig. 1.16

CASE 8

An elderly female patient was referred for a barium swallow to investigate mild dysphagia and progressive, though non-specific, upper gastrointestinal discomfort.

What abnormality is seen in the lower oesophagus on this oblique radiograph (Fig. 1.17) taken from a barium swallow series?

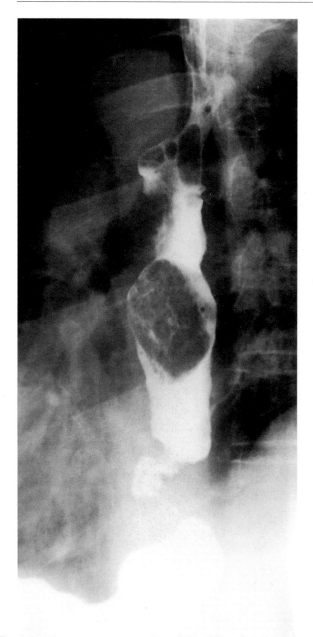

Fig. 1.17

The barium swallow radiograph, oblique projection (Fig. 1.17), shows a well-circumscribed filling defect (5 cm in its long axis) which appears to be expanding into the lumen of the lower oesophagus. A lateral view revealed this lesion to be narrowing the lumen and to be submucosal in origin. The appearances are those of an oesophageal leiomyoma.

Oesophageal leiomyoma

• Usually identified as an incidental finding, though some may present with slowly progressive symptoms.
• Solitary and variable in size up to 8 cm.
• Benign, submucosal tumour.
• Distributed mainly within the lower third of the oesophagus.

The axial postcontrast CT image (Fig. 1.18), taken from a different patient, demonstrates a benign gastric leiomyoma arising from the posterior wall of the stomach and outlined by oral contrast medium (arrow). CT imaging can be very helpful in determining the size and extent of submucosal tumours which may be significantly underestimated by barium studies alone. Benign lesions are usually uniform in texture and are well circumscribed. Malignant degeneration should be suspected in large lesions which enhance inhomogeneously, are of heterogeneous texture and contain calcification.

Further reading

Levine, M.S., Buck J.L., Pantongrag-Brown, L. et al. (1996) Oesophageal leiomyomatosis. Radiology **199**, 533–536.

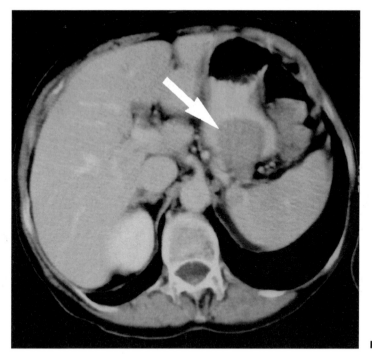

Fig. 1.18

CASE 9

A middle-aged male patient with a previous history of coronary artery bypass surgery had a barium meal examination to investigate symptoms of gastro-oesophageal reflux.

What abnormal features are highlighted in the anteroposterior (AP) radiograph of the stomach (Fig. 1.19)?

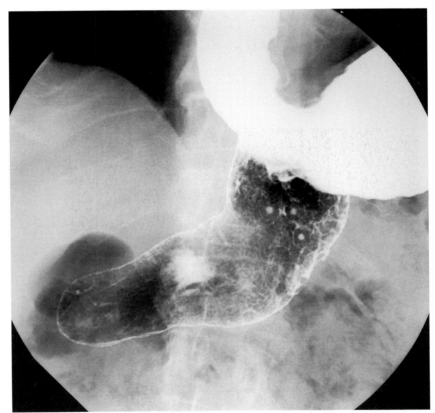

Fig. 1.19

A reproduced, though magnified, view (Fig. 1.20) of the barium meal radiograph demonstrates multiple 'bull's-eye' lesions in the body of the stomach (curved arrows). Multiple polypoid lesions are seen in profile on the greater curve of the stomach (straight arrows) with pools of barium lying in small central ulcers when the polyps are seen *en face*, giving the so-called 'bull's-eye' appearance (curved arrows). The patient also had gastro-oesophageal reflux noted during fluoroscopy.

Differential diagnosis of multiple gastric filling defects

- Hyperplastic polyps.
- Adenomatous polyps.
- Fundic gland polyps.

- 'See-through' artefacts (e.g. phleboliths projected over the stomach).
- Polyposis syndromes.

Endoscopy with biopsy is advised since it is rarely possible to distinguish polyp types radiologically. Most (65–90%) are hyperplastic polyps that are regenerative, non-neoplastic lesions and usually smaller than 2 cm. There is no strong relationship with gastric cancer. In contrast adenomatous polyps are truly premalignant, particularly if larger than 2 cm in diameter.

Further reading

Buck, J.L. & Pantongrag-Brown, L. (1994) Gastritides, gastropathies, and polyps unique to the stomach. *The Radiologic Clinics of North America*, pp. 1215–1231.

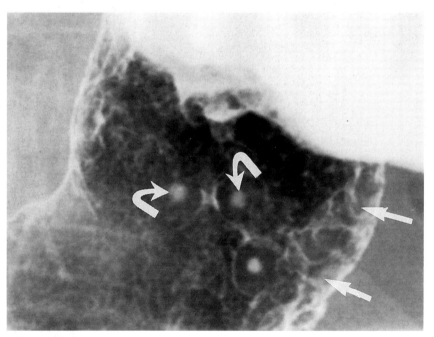

Fig. 1.20

CASE 10

This elderly and frail male patient presented with a history of weight loss, altered bowel habit and blood with mucus per rectum. Co-morbidity included severe peripheral vascular disease, poor left ventricular function and impaired renal function.

What abnormality is shown on this oblique image of the sigmoid colon (Fig. 1.21) taken during a double-contrast barium enema examination? What other imaging tests would you undertake initially and how would these influence your management?

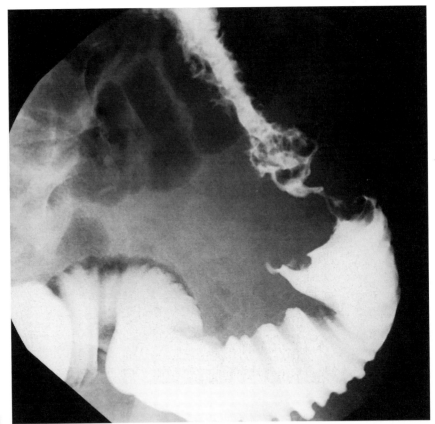

Fig. 1.21

This double-contrast barium enema image (Fig. 1.21) demonstrates an irregular stricture in the distal descending colon with shouldering and mucosal destruction typical of a carcinoma. Histological confirmation was gained by flexible sigmoidoscopy and biopsy.

Further imaging was confined to a chest radiograph and ultrasound scan of the abdomen. The presence of cardiomegaly was confirmed and an ultrasound scan revealed multiple 'target' lesions in the liver consistent with metastases.

This patient has therefore incurable disease and his general poor condition precludes surgical intervention. Considerable risks accompany palliative surgery. An alternative palliative procedure is the insertion of a self-expanding metallic stent (SEMS) per rectum which was undertaken in this patient (Fig. 1.22). An introducing catheter can be seen in the sigmoid colon with a wire crossing the tumour. The deployed stent can be seen *in situ* with a 'waist' (arrow) at the site of stricture.

Advantages of SEMS in the management of malignant large bowel obstruction

- Palliation of symptoms in patients with incurable disease and/or high surgical risk.
- Relief of acute large bowel obstruction prior to accurate preoperative tumour staging.
- Relief of acute large bowel obstruction to allow resuscitation and to optimize the patient's medical condition.

Disadvantages of colonic SEMS

- Failure to relieve obstruction.
- Faecal impaction of stent lumen.
- Tumour ingrowth/overgrowth.
- Tumour rupture with perforation.
- Stent migration.

Further reading

Mainar, A., De Gregorio, M.A., Tejero, E. *et al.* (1999) Acute colorectal obstruction: treatment with self-expanding metal stents before scheduled surgery—results of a multicentre study. *Radiology* **210**, 65–69.

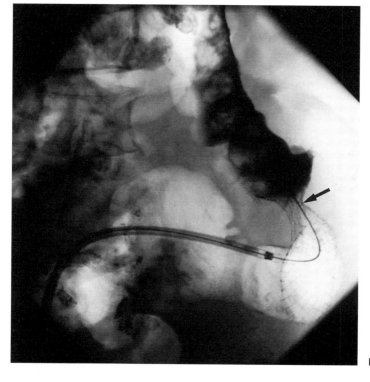

Fig. 1.22

CASE 11

A 73-year-old man presented with progressive, painless jaundice and weight loss. An ultrasound scan demonstrated a normal-calibre common bile duct and normal pancreas, though the intrahepatic ducts were grossly dilated. CT imaging confirmed these findings and demonstrated an ill-defined mass in relation to the porta hepatis.

What examination is illustrated below (Fig. 1.23)?
What abnormality is demonstrated and what is the differential diagnosis?
What alternative imaging techniques could give this information?
Which therapeutic procedures are available and how may a positive diagnosis be obtained?

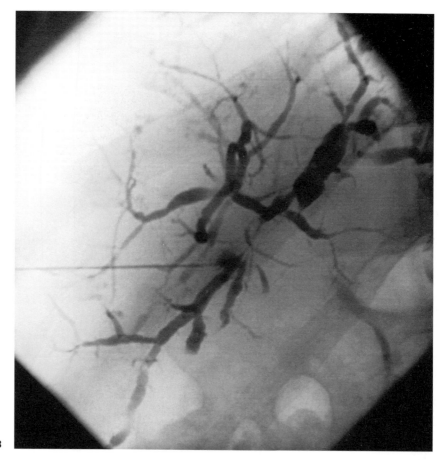

Fig. 1.23

Figure 1.23 is taken from a percutaneous cholan-giogram (PTC). Contrast infusion via a fine-needle right lobe puncture demonstrates extrinsic compression of the confluence of the main intrahepatic bile ducts and the common hepatic duct.

Differential diagnosis of biliary bifurcation obstruction

- Metastases (intrahepatic/nodal).
- Cholangiocarcinoma (the diagnosis in this case).
- Primary liver tumours.
- Inflammatory mass/benign stricture.

CT imaging and MR cholangiography are both helpful in pretherapeutic assessment of hilar lesions. Endoscopic retrograde cholangiopancreatography will also demonstrate the level of obstruction but may not delineate the intrahepatic ducts and therefore the extent of the lesion. Outlining all the intrahepatic ducts at PTC may require left and right lobe punctures.

Malignant hilar obstruction is almost invariably surgically unresectable. Palliation can be gained by percutaneous or endoscopic stenting with the best results being obtained by bilateral drainage using self-expanding metallic stents (SEMS). This was performed in this case and is illustrated in Fig. 1.24 where SEMS (arrows) have been placed in both main hepatic ducts and free flow of contrast into the duodenum has been established.

Percutaneous biopsy and bile cytology are less reliable than endobiliary brush cytology in the confirmation of malignancy.

Further reading

Lee, B.H., Choe, D.H., Lee, J.H., Kim, K.H. & Chin, S.Y. (1997) Metallic stents in malignant biliary obstruction: prospective long-term results. *American Journal of Roentgenology* **168**, 741–745.

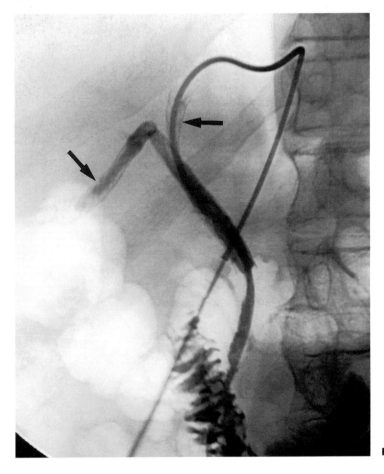

Fig. 1.24

CASE 12

A scheduled colectomy to manage this young adult patient's acute ulcerative colitis was postponed when she developed a painful, swollen left leg. A colour Doppler ultrasound examination was performed of the left common femoral (Fig. 1.25) and right common femoral (Fig. 1.26) veins.

What does this examination show?
What further management would you consider prior to surgery?

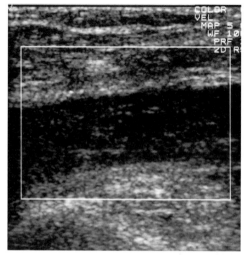

Fig. 1.25

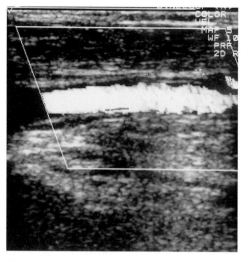

Fig. 1.26

The colour Doppler ultrasound of the left common femoral vein (Fig. 1.25) demonstrates hypoechoic thrombus expanding the lumen of the vessel. The box around the image indicates colour analysis with no flow present. A similar study of the contralateral limb (Fig. 1.26) shows normal flow in a normal-calibre vein on colour Doppler examination.

Ultrasound is currently the initial imaging test of choice for suspected lower limb deep venous thrombosis (DVT). The use of pulsed Doppler allows continuous analysis of the venous waveform. In addition, the compressibility of the vessel under interrogation can be visualized and the flow response to cardiac cycle, respiration and compression of the limb distal may be monitored and compared with the contralateral side. The iliac veins are harder to visualize with ultrasound largely because of overlying bowel gas. If indicated, this segment, as with others, may be imaged by contrast venography, CT or MR imaging.

The surgical management of this patient is complicated by the presence of a proven DVT and added risk of pulmonary embolism. Anticoagulation is contraindicated in the short term and so this patient was managed with a removable (temporary) inferior vena caval (IVC) filter.

IVC filters

Indications for insertion of an IVC filter in the presence of pulmonary embolism or iliofemoral DVT
• Contraindication to anticoagulation.
• Failure of anticoagulation.
• Complications of anticoagulation.

Complications of IVC filters
• Migration.
• Fracture/disintegration.
• Erosion of IVC wall.
• IVC thrombosis.

Further reading

Dorfman, G.S. & Cronan, J.J. (1992) Venous ultrasonography. *The Radiologic Clinics of North America*. W.B. Saunders Co., Philadelphia, pp. 879–892.

CHAPTER 2

Stephen G. Ho and Peter L. Munk

CASE 1

A 45-year-old patient presented complaining of progressive left hip pain over a 2-month period. An anteroposterior (AP) radiograph of the hips (Fig. 2.1) with a lateral view of the left hip (Fig. 2.2) is demonstrated. The patient had previously been healthy with no history of trauma or other painful joints.

What is the diagnosis?
What feature is highlighted in Fig. 2.2?

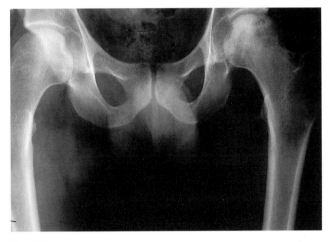

Fig. 2.1

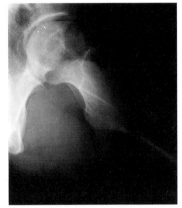

Fig. 2.2

The diagnosis is avascular necrosis of the left femoral head with evidence of early collapse.

The most striking feature of the AP radiograph (Fig. 2.1) is irregularity of the superior aspect of the left femoral head with a large associated area of rarefaction consistent with a subchondral cyst. On the lateral view radiograph (Fig. 2.2) a thin area of radiolucency is noted subcortically (arrows), representing early fracturing.

Key radiological features in avascular necrosis on radiographs

• A subcortical line is one of the earliest radiographic signs and usually precedes collapse.
• The cranial aspect of the femoral head may have a mottled trabecular pattern with accompanying patchy sclerosis, irregularity, flattening and fragmentation.
• In the early phase the acetabular side of the joint appears entirely normal.
• Superimposed degenerative arthritis accompanies the chronic phase.

Often by the time radiographic changes of avascular necrosis are evident, the process is well established and irreversible. Early stage detection is therefore of paramount importance. MR imaging has been proven to be more sensitive than isotope bone scanning and has become the imaging modality of choice in detecting early avascular necrosis. It may also detect early avascular necrosis in the contralateral hip before this becomes clinically symptomatic.

Coronal T1-weighted MR images (Fig. 2.3) from a different patient demonstrate the expected avascular necrosis in the right hip. Additionally there is clearly evidence of changes in the left asymptomatic side. The black line in both femoral heads (arrows) demarcates the normal bone from an avascular segment cranially. The area of higher signal intensity (curved arrows) within the femoral head has been found to correlate with infarcted bone on histological examination.

Further reading

Gabriel, H., Fitzgerald, S.W., Myers, M.T., Donaldson, J.S. & Poznanski, A.K. (1994) MR imaging of hip disorders. *RadioGraphics* **14**, 763–781.

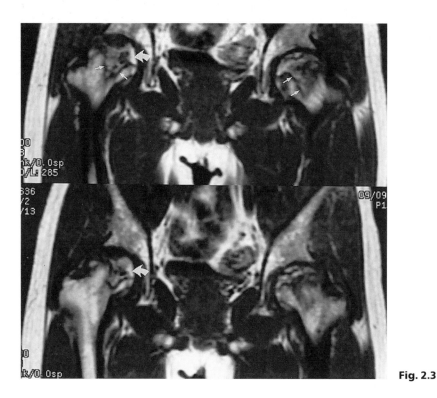

Fig. 2.3

CASE 2

A 9-year-old child presents with a 2-day history of left hip pain and a greatly reduced range of movement. No predisposing medical condition is present or a clear history of trauma. On physical examination the hip is maintained in a flexed and externally rotated position. Movement causes extreme discomfort.

An anteroposterior (AP) radiograph (Fig. 2.4) of the hips was obtained.

What is the most likely diagnosis?
What would you wish to do next?

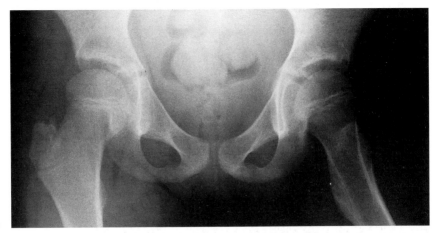

Fig. 2.4

The AP radiograph of the pelvis (Fig. 2.4) indicates that the hip joint space at its medial aspect is slightly wider on the left than the right (widened teardrop sign), a feature suggestive of a joint effusion. Additionally the obturator fat stripe, just medial to the hip within the soft tissues of the pelvis, is clearly seen on the right though absent on the left side. These features are strongly suggestive of an intra-articular inflammatory process. Septic arthritis of the left hip joint must be considered.

The next step should be joint aspiration. Ultrasound not only provides a non-invasive means of demonstrating hip joint effusion but also enables accurate intra-articular needle placement. Alternatively, fluoroscopic guidance may be used.

Septic arthritis

• Common organisms include *Staphyloccus aureus / S. epidermidis*, group B streptococci.
• Localized pain, reduced joint movement and effusion.

• Fever, leucocytosis, elevated erythrocyte sedimentation rate.

Aspirated joint fluid is sent for analysis and culture. Prompt drainage of an infected hip joint gives the highest chance for preservation of joint function. Continuous irrigation and serial aspiration are alternative methods, though each requires systemic antibiotic therapy.

The pelvic radiograph below illustrates the consequences of an unrecognized septic joint (Fig. 2.5). The left femoral head has eroded and collapsed with profound loss of cartilage superiorly. The femur has migrated cranially and laterally.

Osteomyelitis has intervened and is manifested radiologically in both iliac and femoral bones by mottled sclerosis and lysis.

Further reading

Forrester, D.M. & Feske, W.I. (1996) Imaging of infectious arthritis. *Seminars in Roentgenology* **31**, 239–249.

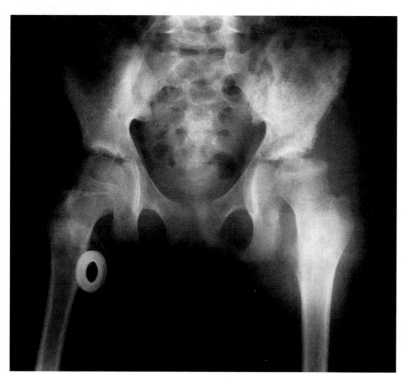

Fig. 2.5

CASE 3

A 21-year-old patient complains of progressively more intense right mid-thigh pain. There is no history of trauma. It seems worse at night and is not aggravated by physical activity.

What abnormal features are evident on the anteroposterior (AP) and lateral radiographs (Figs 2.6 & 2.7, respectively) of the right mid-femur?
What do the arrows highlight?
What clinical diagnosis would you consider? Suggest further imaging that may support this.

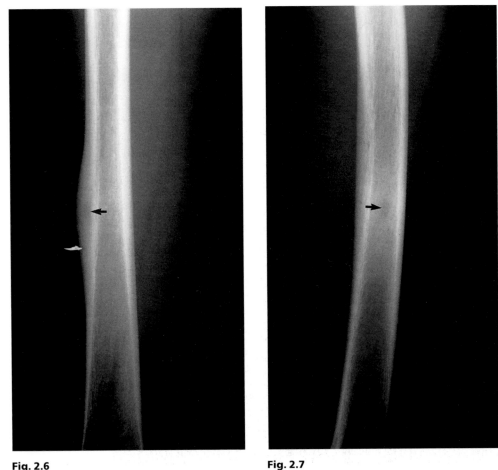

Fig. 2.6   **Fig. 2.7**

The radiographs (Figs 2.6 & 2.7) demonstrate a mature thick periosteal reaction around a longitudinally ovoid area of vague radiolucency (arrows). The diagnosis is osteoid osteoma of the femoral diaphysis. The area of radiolucency (arrows) represents an osteoid osteoma nidus with an intense sclerotic bone reaction surrounding it.

Osteoid osteoma

• Benign bony neoplasm of unknown aetiology.
• Incidence is highest in the second decade but rare in those over the age of 30.
• Commonly located in the tibia and femur; when in the spine it favours the posterior elements.
• Creates a sharp, boring pain which is usually worse at night and often relieved with salicylates.
• Local tenderness, scoliosis, overgrowth of bone or secondary synovitis if located near a joint.

• Lesion cured by complete excision of the nidus. Alternatively image-guided radiofrequency ablation/alcohol injection is used.
• Spontaneous regression may occur, though this often takes months or years.

In this patient the diagnosis was confirmed using radionucleotide bone scanning (Fig. 2.8) which shows an area of increased uptake in the right mid-femur. Axial CT imaging was also performed and demonstrates marked cortical thickening with a central area of radiolucency (the nidus—arrow, Fig. 2.9) which contains a tiny internal calcified region.

Further reading

Rosenthal, D.I., Hornick, F.J., Wolfe, M.N., Jennings, L.C., Gephart, M.C. & Mankin, H.J. (1998) Changes in the management of osteoid osteoma. *Journal of Bone and Joint Surgery* **80A**, 815–821.

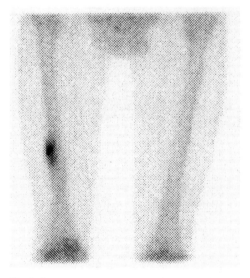

Fig. 2.8

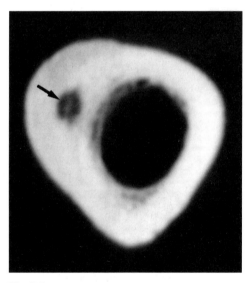

Fig. 2.9

CASE 4

This 35-year-old patient sustained a right posterior hip dislocation at the time of a motor vehicle accident and was admitted to hospital. The dislocation was reduced and an anteroposterior (AP) radiograph (Fig. 2.10) of the right hip was obtained.

What abnormality is highlighted on the radiograph?

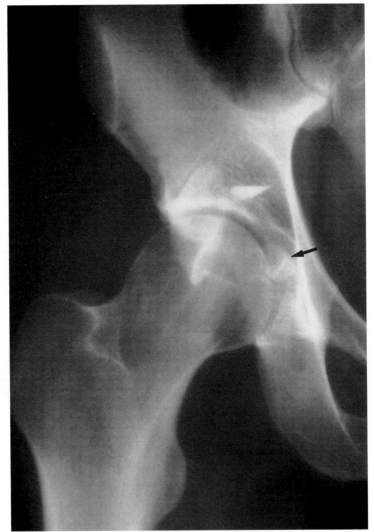

Fig. 2.10

The AP radiograph of the right hip (Fig. 2.10) demonstrates irregularity to the posterior rim of the acetabulum consistent with a history of a posterior hip dislocation and marginal fracture. A trapped intra-articular fragment is highlighted.

Posterior dislocation of the hip

• Typical injury during head-on motor vehicle collision where the knee impacts against the dashboard.
• Associated fracture of the posterior rim is common.
• During the process of reduction an osseous fragment will be trapped intra-articularly.
• Small fragments (less than 0.5 cm) may be impossible to detect on plain radiographs.
• Degenerative changes often develop even without trapped fragments.

CT imaging may be invaluable because it allows detection of fragments as small as 2 mm in size. An axial CT image (Fig. 2.11) taken of a different patient following left posterior hip dislocation clearly illustrates the presence of a small fragment in the left hip joint (arrow). Note the deficiency in the posterior rim of the acetabulum consistent with the fracture produced by the posterior dislocation. MR imaging is a useful adjunct in the assessment of soft tissue trauma, e.g. sciatic nerve injury, produced by posterior hip dislocation.

Further reading

Potter, H.G., Montgomery, K.D., Heise, C.W. & Helfet, D.L. (1993) MR imaging of acetabular fractures: value of detecting femoral head injury, intra-articular fragments, and sciatic nerve injury. *American Journal of Roentgenology* **163**, 881–886.

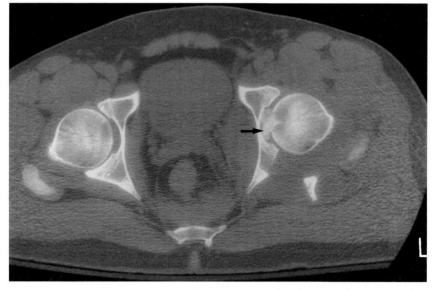

Fig. 2.11

CASE 5

A 47-year-old male complains of throbbing left thigh pain which has worsened over a period of months. The symptoms are poorly localized and unrelated to activity.

What abnormal radiological features are present in the lateral radiograph (Fig. 2.12) of the left lower femur?
What is your diagnosis?

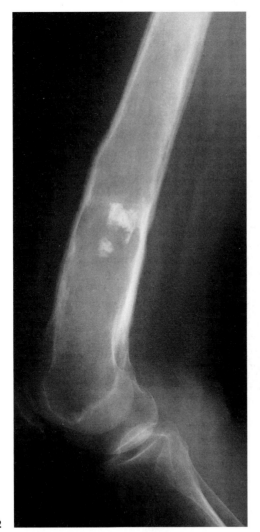

Fig. 2.12

The lateral radiograph (Fig. 2.12) demonstrates an expansile lesion within the distal left femoral diaphysis and metaphysis producing endosteal scalloping. Areas of coarse calcification can be visualized within the lesion. These radiographic appearances are consistent with a cartilaginous tumour, and biopsy confirmed the diagnosis of chondrosarcoma. Differentiating enchondroma from chondrosarcoma can be difficult. Features indicative of chondrosarcoma include large size (> 5 cm), pain related to the lesion, extensive endosteal scalloping, frank cortical destruction in the presence of a soft tissue mass and periosteal reaction.

Chondrosarcoma

- Most are enostotic.
- Occurs principally in adults.
- Predilection for long bones and rare below the knees and elbows.
- Centrally placed and located in the metaphysis or diaphysis (or both).
- Treatment invariably requires surgery with more radical excision for high-grade lesions.

As a general principle in evaluation of intramedullary bone tumours, the entire length of the bone should be evaluated to rule out possible skip-lesions. These are particularly common with Ewing's sarcoma and osteosarcoma, less so with chondrosarcoma.

MR imaging often demonstrates lesions to be more extensive than is apparent on radiographs. This case is no exception. Sagittal MR images of the lower left femur (Fig. 2.13) reveal that the lesion extends further distally, adjacent to the margin of the joint. The tumour is seen as high-signal material within the femur (arrows) and contains central areas of low signal corresponding to areas of calcification seen on the radiograph (curved arrows). This is invaluable information in therapeutic planning, since a joint-sparing procedure would not have been adequate in this case.

Further reading

Springfield, D.S., Gebhardt, M.C. & McGuire, M.H. (1996) Chondrosarcoma: A review. *Journal of Bone and Joint Surgery* **78A**, 141–149.

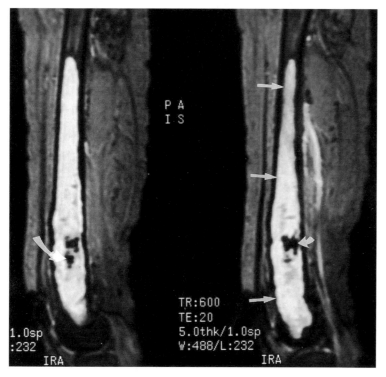

Fig. 2.13

CASE 6

A 35-year-old rugby football player sustained an acute knee injury which resulted in temporary swelling of the joint. However, some weeks later he presented with pain and instability of the knee during activities. On physical examination the knee looked normal. There was no specific tenderness, though he was reluctant to allow full range of movement. The Lachman test (lifting the tibia forward on the femur) was positive, indicating increased ligamentous laxity.

T1-weighted MR images (Fig. 2.14) were obtained of the knee in both sagittal and oblique sagittal planes.

What is the diagnosis?

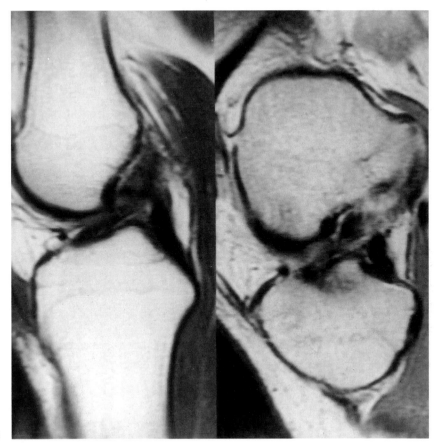

Fig. 2.14

This patient has sustained a tear of the anterior cruciate ligament. The normally straight, virtually parallel fibres of the anterior cruciate ligament are noted to be grossly disrupted and poorly defined. This becomes more apparent when contrasted with a comparable MR image (Fig. 2.15) of a normal anterior cruciate ligament (arrows).

Anterior cruciate ligament

• Arises from the anterior tibial spine and runs obliquely and superiorly to attach to the medial side of the lateral femoral condyle.
• Intra-articular but extrasynovial.
• Prevents anterior tibial translation and posterior displacement of the femur with knee flexion.

• Does not heal or become functional after disruption.
• Distribution is frequently accompanied by injuries to the menisci, capsule and other intra-articular structures.

MR imaging has been shown to be highly accurate in the evaluation of disorders of the anterior cruciate ligament and is the initial imaging modality of choice.

Further reading

Lee, J.K., Yao, L., Phelps, C.T., Wirth, C.R., Czajka, J. & Loxman, J. (1988) Anterior cruciate ligament tears: MR imaging compared with arthroscopy and clinical tests. *Radiology* **166**, 861–864.

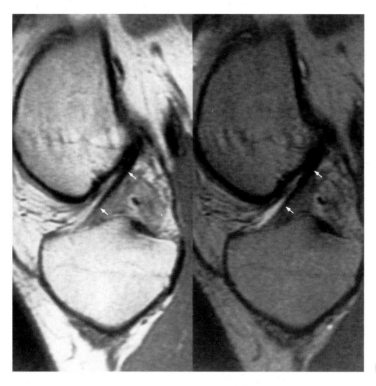

Fig. 2.15

CASE 7

A 75-year-old female presented as an emergency with abdominal pain and distension. On examination, the abdomen was distended and diffusely tender. No hernias were present. High-pitched bowel sounds were audible. Rectal examination revealed an empty rectum.

What abnormal features are present on the supine abdominal radiograph (Fig. 2.16)?
What is the diagnosis?

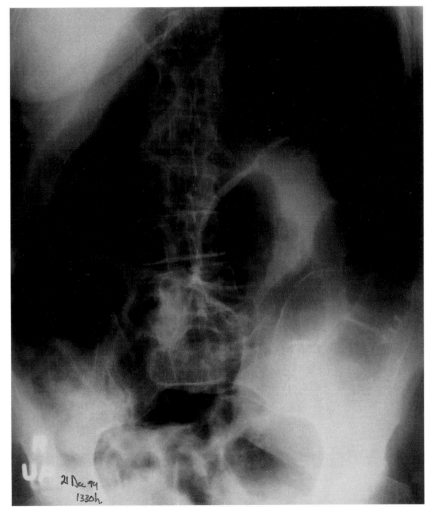

Fig. 2.16

The abdominal radiograph (Fig. 2.16) shows a massively dilated loop of bowel with an inverted U, or coffee-bean, appearance directed towards the left upper quadrant. Its 'axis' is directed towards the pelvis. There are absent haustral markings in this loop which measures approximately 10 cm in diameter. Colonic bowel gas is also identified along the distribution of the descending colon. Multiple dilated loops of small bowel are present throughout the abdomen.

These features are in keeping with a closed loop obstruction due to sigmoid volvulus. This was confirmed by a low-pressure water-soluble contrast enema (Fig. 2.17). This demonstrates a smooth, tapered beaking of the colon at the rectosigmoid junction (arrow).

Volvulus of the sigmoid colon

• Common in the African and Asian continents.

• Related to high dietary fibre, acquired megacolon, chronic constipation.
• In Europe and North America patients are usually elderly, institutionalized or suffering from psychiatric and chronic neurological diseases.
• Initial management with endoscopic deflation (rigid sigmoidoscopy and passage of flatus tube) is often successful, though recurrence rates are high.
• Sigmoid resection and exteriorization carry a significant mortality rate despite appropriate preoperative resuscitation.

Further reading

Ballantyne, G.H. (1982) Review of sigmoid volvulus: clinical patterns and pathogenesis. *Diseases of the Colon and Rectum* **25**, 823–830.

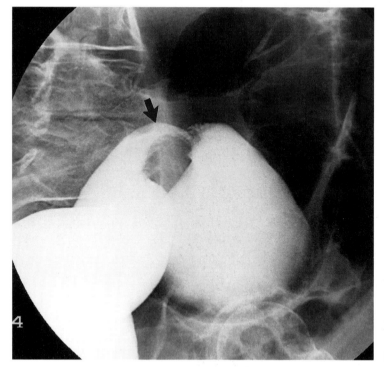

Fig. 2.17

CASE 8

A 45-year-old female presents with recurrent mid-abdominal pain. She has a history of alcohol abuse.

A magnified radiograph of the epigastric region is performed (Fig. 2.18).

What further investigations has the patient had (Fig. 2.19)?
What abnormalities are present?
What is the diagnosis?

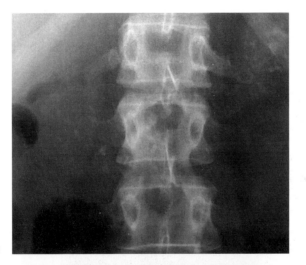

Fig. 2.18

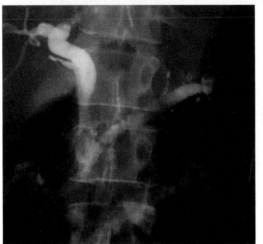

Fig. 2.19

The upper abdominal radiograph (Fig. 2.18) demonstrates punctate calcification in the epigastrium in an oblique distribution towards the left upper quadrant. The features were diagnostic for chronic calcific pancreatitis. The second image (Fig. 2.19) has been obtained from an endoscopic retrograde cholangiopancreatography (ERCP) examination.

The reproduced ERCP image (Fig. 2.20) shows several of the features of chronic pancreatitis. There is dilatation of the main pancreatic duct with dilatation of several side branches (curved arrows) and there is loss of the normal tapering of the main pancreatic duct peripherally. No focal stenoses are seen. However, a rounded intraluminal filling defect is present (arrow), representing an intraductal calculus.

ERCP changes of chronic pancreatitis

• Earliest changes involve first- and second-order side branches of the main pancreatic duct.
• Side-branch dilatation, clubbing and stenosis occur.

• Main pancreatic duct involvement is seen in advanced disease with dilatation, stenosis and calculus formation.
• Stenoses are usually short and smooth, unlike those seen in neoplasm.

ERCP is a useful though invasive technique in the diagnosis of chronic pancreatitis. It can give rise to complications which, on rare occasions, prove fatal. MR cholangiopancreatography does provide a useful, non-invasive alternative. Ultrasound and CT are also both useful in assessing size and contour of the pancreas, dilatation and shape of the pancreatic duct, and the presence of ductal calcifications.

Further reading

Radecki, P.D., Friedman, A.C. & Dabezies, M.A. (1994) Pancreatitis. In: *Radiology of the Liver, Biliary Tract, and Pancreas* (eds A.C. Friedman & A.H. Dachman), pp. 763–805. Mosby-Year Book, St Louis, Missouri.

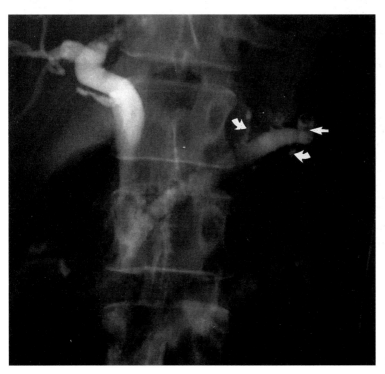

Fig. 2.20

CHAPTER 2

CASE 9

A 73-year-old male presented with acute-on-chronic right lower abdominal pain. This was accompanied by a long history of intermittent, watery and often blood-stained diarrhoea. Abdominal examination revealed local tenderness in the right mid- to lower abdomen with the suspicion of an accompanying mass. Active bowel sounds were heard throughout the abdomen.

What investigation is depicted in the radiograph (Fig. 2.21)?
What is the diagnosis?
Describe the radiological abnormalities that support this.

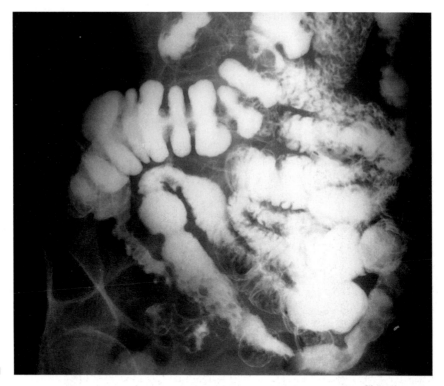

Fig. 2.21

The radiograph (Fig. 2.21) is part of a series from a barium examination of the small bowel.

This patient has Crohn's disease.

Crohn's disease

Differential diagnosis of Crohn's disease
• Acute: infective causes, e.g. *Yersinia enterocolitica*.
• Chronic: lymphoma, Behçet's disease, tuberculosis, actinomycosis and adenocarcinoma.

Key radiological features (highlighted in Fig. 2.22) are those of luminal narrowing, patchy asymmetrical involvement (open arrows) and small deep fissures seen in the terminal ileum (arrows). No distinct fistulae are identified and the disease appears to be limited to the distal ileum. The caecum and ascending colon are spared. There is separation of distal small bowel loops secondary to wall thickening and oedema.

Features of Crohn's disease on small bowel barium studies
• Lymphoid follicle hyperplasia is an early sign of disease.
• Aphthous ulceration.
• Fold thickening.
• 'Rose-thorn' ulceration.
• Inflammatory pseudopolyps.
• Transmural fissures are seen in advanced disease ('cobblestone' appearance).
• Complications include strictures, abscess formation and fistulae. Moreover, there is an increased incidence of small bowel malignancy.

Further reading

Wills, J.S., Lobis, I.F. & Denstman, F.J. (1997) Crohn disease. State of the art. *Radiology* **202**, 597–610.

Crohn, B.B., Ginzburg, L. & Oppenheimer, G.D. (1932) Regional ileitis: a pathological clinical entity. *Journal of the American Medical Association* **99**, 1323–1329.

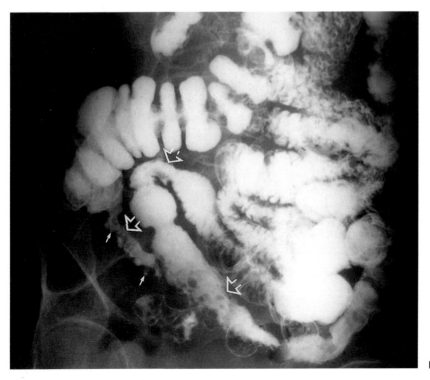

Fig. 2.22

CASE 10

A 58-year-old female presents with chronic episodic right upper quadrant abdominal pain. Punctate calcification is identified in the wall of the gall bladder on this axial CT image (Fig. 2.23) of the right upper quadrant. No definite gallstone was identified.

What is the diagnosis?
What is the next step in management?

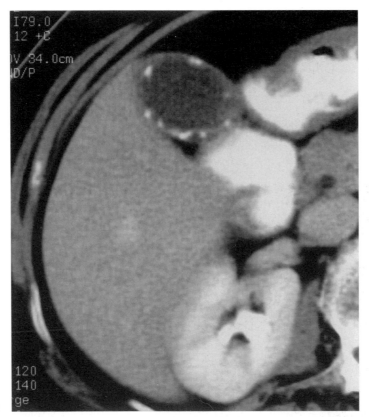

Fig. 2.23

The calcification of the gallbladder wall is termed 'porcelain gall bladder'.

On the reproduced axial CT image (Fig. 2.24) calcifications can be seen in the gallbladder wall as areas of high attenuation (arrows). The gall bladder contains low-attenuation bile. Oral contrast is seen in adjacent duodenum (curved arrow).

Calcification of the gallbladder wall ('porcelain gall bladder')

- Rare condition, female predominance.
- Calcification may be punctuate or continuous.
- Cholelithiasis is commonly evident.
- Reflects end-stage chronic cholecystitis.
- Associated with a high frequency of gallbladder carcinoma.

As there is a significant association (12.5–60%) between porcelain gall bladder and gallbladder carcinoma, the next recommended step in management would be cholecystectomy.

Gallbladder cancer has a poor prognosis with an overall 5-year survival rate of little more than 5%. Radical surgical resection does not achieve significant improvement in outcome and adjuvant therapy is ineffective. Limited disease may be managed by simple cholecystectomy with postoperative radiation therapy. Palliative cholecystectomy and an accompanying biliary bypass procedure, where possible, are indicated for extensive disease.

Further reading

Shimizu, M., Miura, J., Tanaka, T. *et al.* (1989) Porcelain gallbladder: relation between its type by ultrasound and incidence of cancer. *Journal of Clinical Gastroenterology* **11**, 471–476.

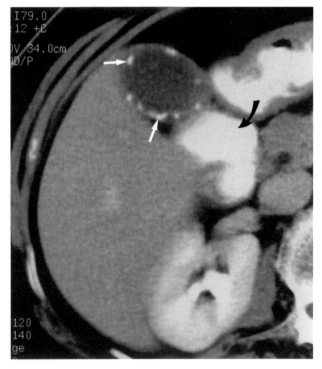

Fig. 2.24

CASE 11

An 87-year-old male presented with acute abdominal pain. Physical examination revealed a rigid abdomen. An erect chest radiograph was performed (Fig. 2.25).

What is the diagnosis?

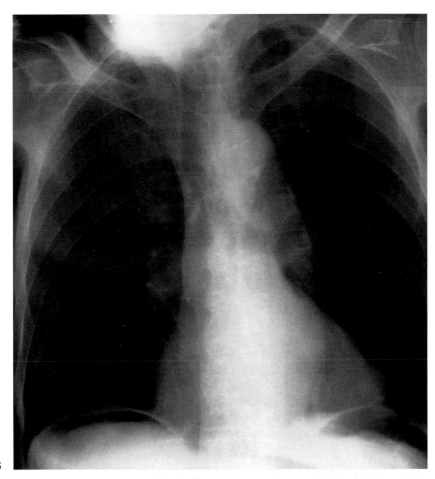

Fig. 2.25

The erect chest radiograph (Fig. 2.25) reveals free subdiaphragmatic, intraperitoneal air. The diagnostic feature is the presence of curvilinear gas lucency under both hemidiaphragms.

Differential diagnosis of free intraperitoneal air

- Perforated viscus: inflammation infarction or neoplasm.
- Iatrogenic: recent surgery or peritoneal dialysis.
- Accompanying pneumothorax or pneumomediastinum.
- Ruptured cysts from pneumatosis cystoides intestinalis.

An upper gastrointestinal contrast study was performed using a water-soluble medium. An image (Fig. 2.26) from this series demonstrates free spillage of contrast from the duodenal bulb into the peritoneal space (arrows).

The presence of pneumoperitoneum in an acutely ill patient demands active resuscitation prior to a laparotomy. An anterior perforated duodenal ulcer is the most common cause. Ulcers may also perforate posteriorly. Gas is then confined to the retroperitoneum and may not be evident on radiographs. Indeed, up to 30% of peptic ulcer perforations do not reveal evidence of free subdiaphragmatic, intraperitoneal air.

Further reading

Levine, M.S. (1994) Peptic ulcers. In: *Textbook of Gastrointestinal Radiology* (eds R.M. Gore, M.S. Levine & I. Laufer). W.B. Saunders Co., Philadelphia, pp. 587–589.

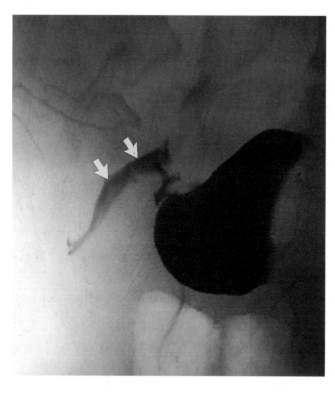

Fig. 2.26

CASE 12

An elderly male presents as an emergency with abdominal pain and vomiting. A long-standing, right inguinal hernia is only partly controlled by an external support (truss). The hernia proves irreducible on physical examination.

What does the supine abdominal radiograph show (Fig. 2.27) show?

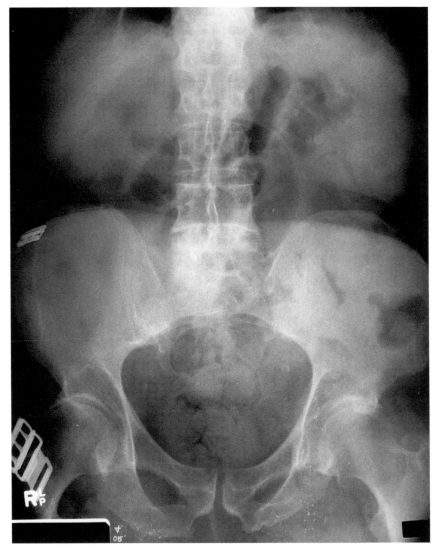

Fig. 2.27

The supine abdominal radiograph (Fig. 2.27) demonstrates several dilated central loops of small bowel. Gas and stool are identified in the rectum. A rounded calcific density is projected over the lower aspect of the right sacroiliac joint. Gas lucency can be seen projected over the right obturator foramen representing air within the hernia sac. The radiological features are consistent with small bowel obstruction due to incarceration of this hernia.

A further supine radiograph (Fig. 2.28) shows a grossly enlarged scrotum containing loops of gas-filled bowel. The previously described calcification, representing a calcified mesenteric lymph node, has now fallen into the right hemiscrotum. These features reflect a large inguinal scrotal hernia.

Definitions relating to hernia sac contents

Reducible
Entire hernia sac contents may be returned to the abdominal cavity.

Irreducible
Incomplete reduction of hernia sac contents:

incarcerated—contents are viable;
strangulated—contents may be ischaemic or necrotic.

Sliding
Abdominal viscera form part of the hernia sac wall, i.e. bladder, caecum or sigmoid colon.

Richter's hernia
Only part of the intestinal wall is contained within the hernia without compromise to the lumen. The contained portion of the wall may become strangulated in the absence of intestinal destruction.

Maydl's hernia
The contents of the hernia include two adjacent loops of small bowel with strangulation of the middle segment.

Littre's hernia
A hernia containing a Meckel's diverticulum.

Further reading

Devlin, H.D. (1988) *Management of Abdominal Hernias*. Butterworth & Co., London.

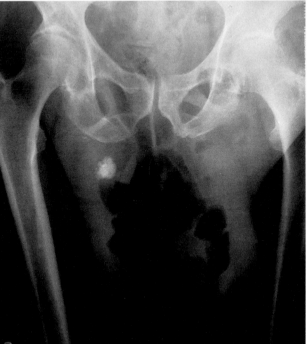

Fig. 2.28

CHAPTER 3

David C. Howlett

CASE 1

A 50-year-old female presents with a 1-week history of fever and left iliac fossa pain. She has had a hysterectomy for endometrial carcinoma 1 month previously.

What abnormalities are evident on the abdominal radiograph (Fig. 3.1)? What other investigations are indicated?

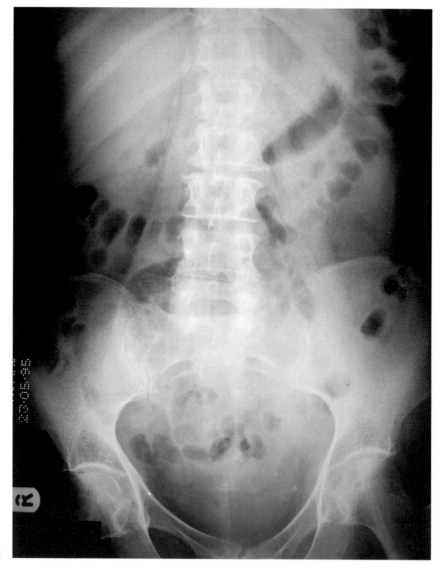

Fig. 3.1

The abdominal radiograph (Fig. 3.1) shows evidence of air within the left iliopsoas muscle seen as streaky linear lucencies in the paravertebral portion. The fat plane along the lateral aspect of the iliopsoas is preserved. Air can be seen tracking down the muscle medial to the left femoral neck before its lesser trochanteric insertion. The appearances are suspicious for air within a psoas abscess. No bony destruction or discitis is evident to provide a clue as to its aetiology.

Ultrasound may provide further information, though views can be limited by overlying bowel gas. CT is the investigation of choice (Fig. 3.2). A fluid collection containing air in the left psoas muscle is demonstrated (arrow) which was subsequently drained percutaneously under CT guidance. A mixed growth of anaerobic bacteria was cultured.

Some causes of iliopsoas compartment involvement

Infection
Infection arises from:
• retroperitoneal organs including kidney;

• the spine following osteomyelitis or discitis, e.g. tuberculosis;
• the gastrointestinal tract, e.g. Crohn's disease, appendicitis;
• pelvic sepsis (as in this case).
    Note: once sepsis penetrates the muscle fascia it may track down into the groin, presenting as an abscess.

Haemorrhage
• In patients with a coagulopathy or on excessive anticoagulant therapy.
• Post-traumatic.
• In patients with leaking aortic aneurysm.

Neoplasia
• Primary, e.g. retroperitoneal sarcoma.
• Secondary, e.g. lymphoma, metastasis.

Further reading

Wegener, O.H. (1992) The retroperitoneal cavity. In: *Whole Body Computed Tomography*, 2nd edn, pp. 451–487. Blackwell Scientific Publications, Oxford.

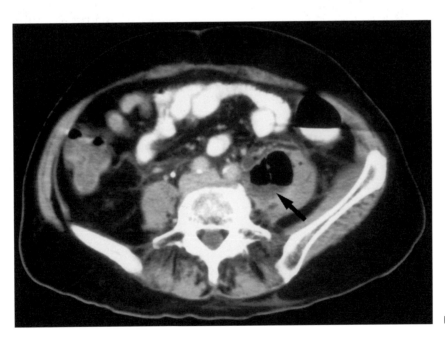

Fig. 3.2

CASE 2

A 55-year-old female presents with a 6-month history of gradual right-sided hearing loss. T1-weighted MR imaging, with contrast enhancement, of the internal auditory canals was performed (Fig. 3.3).

What abnormality is demonstrated?

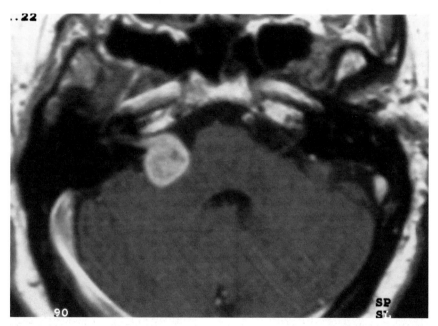

Fig. 3.3

An axial T1-weighted postgadolinium MR examination of the internal auditory canals (IACs) is shown (Fig. 3.3). On a magnified view (Fig. 3.4) an enhancing mass in the right cerebello-pontine angle (large arrow) extends into the right IAC (curved arrow). The intracanalicular portions of the facial and vestibulocochlear nerves can be visualized (small arrows).

The appearances are those of a vestibular schwannoma (VS), also known as acoustic neuroma, which is the commonest cause of a cerebello-pontine angle mass. These are benign nerve sheath tumours which arise from the vestibular nerve. Typically a portion of the tumour extends to, or arises within, the IAC which does allow differentiation from other extra-axial cerebello-pontine angle masses.

Other cerebello-pontine angle lesions

- Meningioma.
- Metastasis.
- Epidermoid.
- Arachnoid cyst.
- Paraganglionoma.
- Chordoma.

When small and intracanalicular, VS tends to adopt the shape of the IAC and to enhance homogeneously following gadolinium administration. Larger lesions protrude into the cerebello-pontine angle and may have an 'ice-cream cone' configuration (Fig. 3.4). Very large lesions may exhibit cystic, haemorrhagic or calcific elements and cause brainstem compression. Bilateral VS occurs in patients with neurofibromatosis type 2 and there is often a family history.

Further reading

Wayne Slone, H. *et al.* (1999) Temporal bone. In: *Magnetic Resonance Imaging* (eds D. Stark & W. Bradley), 3rd edn, pp. 1715–1729. Mosby Inc, St Louis, Missouri.

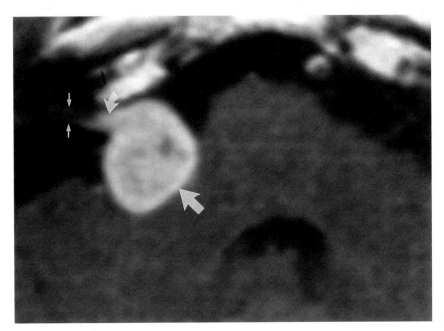

Fig. 3.4

CASE 3

A double-contrast barium enema was performed on this 25-year-old man as part of the investigations into his persistent left lumbar pain. A rigid sigmoidoscopy had revealed multiple polyps, creating a 'carpet-like' appearance in the rectum, some of which were biopsied.

What does this radiograph (Fig. 3.5) from the barium enema series show? What is the diagnosis?

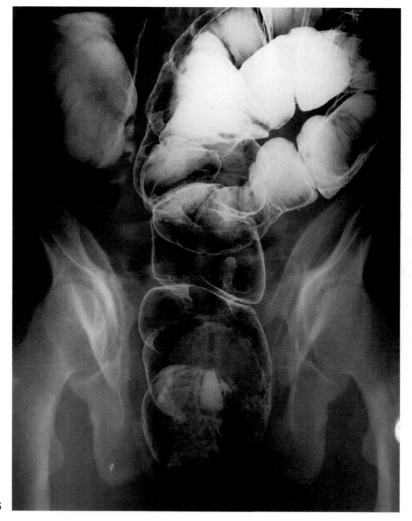

Fig. 3.5

The image from the barium enema series (Fig. 3.5) reveals multiple, widely spread polyps within the rectum and sigmoid colon. Similar features were present throughout the remaining colon. Histology from the rectal biopsy recorded adenomatous change.

This patient has familial adenomatous polyposis (FAP). FAP is inherited in an autosomal dominant manner and is characterized by the presence of hundreds of adenomatous polyps in the large bowel. It is due to an abnormality of the adenomatous polyposis coli (*APC*) gene on chromosome 5q21.

The lumbar symptoms were pursued with postcontrast CT imaging (Fig. 3.6). An enhancing mass in the left quadratus lumborum muscle (arrow) was evident. Histology characterized this to be a desmoid tumour.

Extracolonic manifestations of FAP

• Desmoid tumours (10% incidence in FAP): benign but locally invasive fibromatous tumours prone to recurrence after local resection and most frequently found in relation to the abdominal wall or mesentery.
• Upper gastrointestinal, periampullary and pancreatic carcinomas.
• Thyroid (papillary) carcinoma.
• Medulloblastoma.
• Osteomas.
• Congenital hypertrophy of the retinal pigmented epithelium.

Gardner's syndrome is characterized, in the presence of FAP, by multiple skin lesions, osteomas, desmoid tumours and upper gastrointestinal malignancies.

Further reading

Harned, R.K., Buck, J.L., Olmsted, W.W., Moser, R.P. & Ros, P.R. (1991) Extracolonic manifestations of the familial adenomatous polyposis syndromes. *American Journal of Roentgenology* **156**, 481–485.

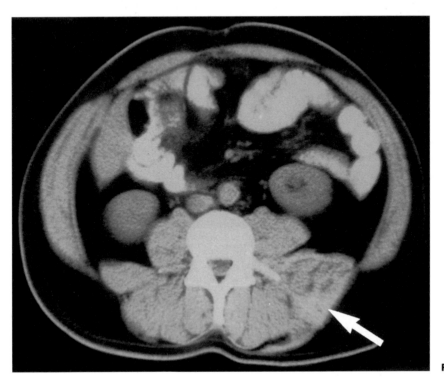

Fig. 3.6

CASE 4

A 16-year-old female presented with chronic bilateral leg swelling and generalized, intermittent abdominal pain and was found to have a reduced serum albumin.

What does the small bowel barium study (Fig. 3.7) demonstrate?
What previous investigation has the patient had?
What is the diagnosis?

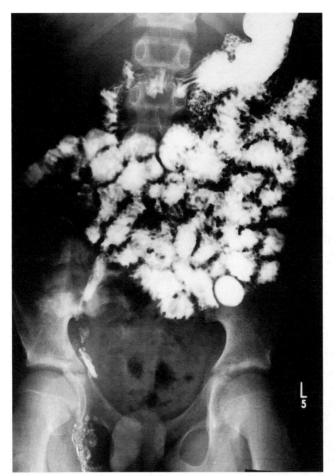

Fig. 3.7

The small bowel barium study film demonstrates diffuse, smooth thickening of the folds of the proximal small bowel (the valvulae conniventes) though the lumen is of normal calibre (Fig. 3.7). Residual contrast is noted within the right femoral and iliac nodes as a result of previous lymphangiography—the clue to the underlying diagnosis.

This patient has a congenital form of lymphangiectasia. Malformation with abnormal dilatation of lymphatics in the villi of the small bowel causes the changes seen (Fig. 3.7). A protein-losing enteropathy may occur due to rupture of dilated lymphatic channels in the gut and also secondary to protein exudation from intestinal capillaries and this causes smooth thickening of the small bowel folds. Atresia of the thoracic duct and hypoplasia of the lower limb lymphatics can also arise.

- *Congenital lymphangiectasia*: young age group and predominantly female.
- *Acquired lymphangiectasia*: secondary to:
  lymphatic obstruction;
  retroperitoneal fibrosis or carcinomatosis;
  diffuse small bowel lymphoma;
  following previous nodal surgery or radiotherapy;
  constrictive pericarditis.

A jejunal biopsy demonstrates distended lymphatics in villi. Multiple biopsies may be needed as these changes may be patchy.

Radiolabelled indirect lymphoscintigraphy is probably the best currently available technique for functional evaluation of the lymphatic system. Radiolabelled tracer is injected subdermally between the toes and lymphatic transport of the macromolecule is tracked with a gamma camera. Tracer disappearance from the foot and accumulation in nodes can be quantified and this technique allows assessment of lymphatic function and visualization of major lymphatic trunks and lymph nodes.

MR lymphangiography has shown promising initial results.

Figure 3.8 shows an image from a technetium-99m lymphoscintigram series in a young female with suspected congenital lymphoedema of the left leg. Sequential images were obtained following injection of nanocolloid into the first web space of both feet. A static image is demonstrated at the level of the thigh and pelvis and normal lymphatic drainage in the right thigh is indicated (arrows). Note is made of normal crossover of lymphatic drainage to the left side with the left femoral and iliac chains demonstrated (open arrows). There is absence of lymphatic drainage within the left limb.

Further reading

Szuba, A. & Rockson, S.G. (1998) Lymphedema: classification, diagnosis and therapy. *Vascular Medicine* **3**, 145–156.

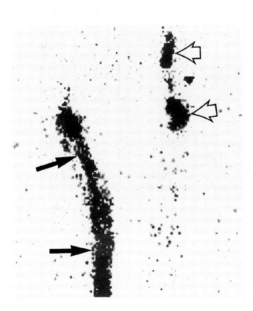

Fig. 3.8

CASE 5

A 22-year-old male presents with acute, generalized abdominal pain.

What abnormalities are apparent on the abdominal radiograph (Fig. 3.9) that might lead towards a diagnosis?
Why may the patient have pain?

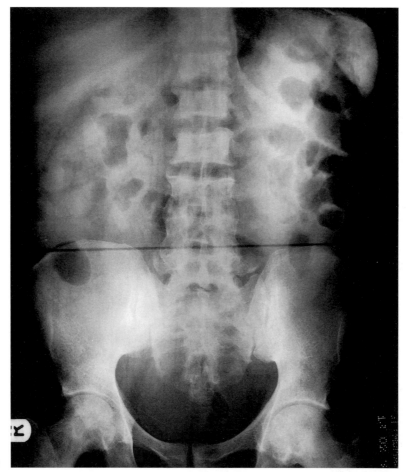

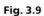

Fig. 3.9

Several abnormalities are present on the abdominal radiograph (Fig. 3.9):
• the spleen is calcified;
• the bony texture is generally coarse with a prominent trabecular pattern;
• there is loss of vertebral end-plate height at several levels in the lumbar spine ('H-type' configuration);
• there is subchondral lucency and sclerosis within the femoral heads.

The diagnosis is sickle-cell disease (SCD). The clinical manifestations of SCD are due to poor solubility of sickle haemoglobin on deoxygenation, when red cells become deformed, assuming a sickle shape. These sickle cells tend to sludge in small blood vessels, causing infarction. The red cell fragility leads to chronic haemolysis and anaemia. Infarction, calcification and bone marrow hyperplasia account for the radiological features observed (Fig. 3.9).

Abdominal pain in SCD

Abdominal pain in SCD may result from:
• gallstones (pigmented due to chronic haemolysis);
• microinfarcts in the gut;
• splenic enlargement secondary to extra-medullary haematopoiesis;
• recurrent splenic microinfarcts causing a reduction in size and calcification as shown on CT imaging (Fig. 3.10, arrow);
• hepatic infarcts and haemosiderosis secondary to multiple blood transfusions which can eventually cause hepatic cirrhosis.

Further reading

Howlett, D.C., Hatrick, A.G., Jarosz, J.M., Bingham, J.B., Cox, T.C. & Irvine, A.T. (1997) The role of CT and MR in imaging the complications of sickle cell disease. *Clinical Radiology* **51**, 821–829.

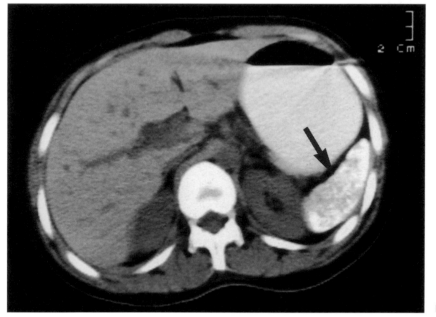

Fig. 3.10

CASE 6

A 22-year-old female presents with a 4-month history of a painless, fluctuant swelling in the anterior triangle of her right neck.

What does postcontrast CT (Fig. 3.11) of the neck demonstrate?
What is the diagnosis?

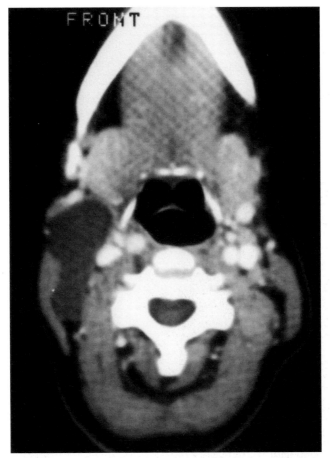

Fig. 3.11

The reproduced CT image (Fig. 3.12) shows a well-circumscribed cystic mass of homogeneous low attenuation in the patient's right neck (white arrow). This deviates the right submandibular gland anteromedially (black arrow), the sterno-cleidomastoid muscle posterolaterally (curved arrow) and the carotid sheath vessels postero-medially (small black arrows).

The appearances (Figs 3.11 & 3.12) are those of a second branchial cleft cyst. Alternative diagnoses to consider in cystic swellings at the angle of the mandible include cystic hygroma, ranula, suppurative lymphadenopathy and subman-dibular sepsis or mucocele.

Branchial cleft abnormalities

• First branchial cleft cysts arise in relation to the parotid gland.
• The second branchial cleft apparatus involutes by the ninth fetal week. Failure of involution allows remnant tissue to develop which may become symptomatic in infants or young adults.

• Ninety-five per cent arise from the remnant of the second branchial apparatus.
• Third branchial cleft cysts are rare and present as a fluctuant swelling in the posterior triangle of the neck.

Ultrasound is useful for initial evaluation of a suspected second branchial cleft cyst, con-firming its cystic nature, although frequently these lesions appear complex, containing haem-orrhagic elements and debris. They may also be associated with a sinus or fistula to the skin enabling secondary infection to intervene.

MR/CT imaging will not only confirm the cys-tic nature of the mass but also delineate the deep extent of the lesion.

Further reading

Harnsberger, H.R. (1995) Cystic masses of the head and neck. In: *Handbook of Head and Neck Imaging*, 2nd edn, pp. 199–223. Mosby Inc, St Louis, Missouri.

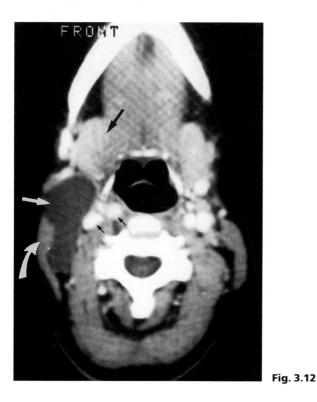

Fig. 3.12

CASE 7

A 68-year-old female presents with a rapidly enlarging, painless right lobe of thyroid. Ultrasound of the thyroid obtained axial images of an abnormal right lobe (Fig. 3.13) and normal left lobe (Fig. 3.14).

What abnormality is evident (Fig. 3.13)?
What diagnosis should be considered?
What further investigations are indicated?

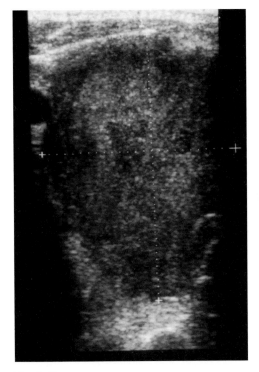

Fig. 3.13

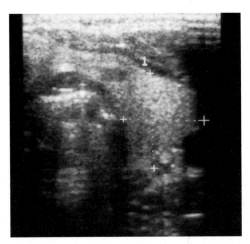

Fig. 3.14

These ultrasound scans demonstrate a large solid mass replacing the right lobe of thyroid gland (Fig. 3.13, cursors) as compared with a normal left lobe (Fig. 3.14, cursors).

Differential diagnosis of solitary, solid thyroid nodule

- Adenoma.
- Haemorrhage into a thyroid cyst.
- Thyroid carcinoma.
- Thyroid lymphoma.
- Metastasis.

Under ultrasound control, core biopsy was performed, the histology of which revealed anaplastic thyroid carcinoma.

Anaplastic thyroid carcinoma accounts for 10–15% of thyroid malignancies. It is characterized by its rapid enlargement, local invasion and early dissemination, often presenting with cervical node involvement. Treatment is limited and usually palliative. The prognosis is poor.

Ultrasound

Ultrasound is the initial imaging modality of choice for palpable thyroid abnormalities. It can:

- determine whether a palpable nodule is solitary or part of a multinodular goitre;
- characterize nodules as cystic or solid;
- identify microcalcifications in malignant solid nodules;
- demonstrate enlarged cervical nodes;
- guide fine-needle aspiration or core biopsy of solid lesions.

CT/MR imaging

CT/MR imaging is used to:
- evaluate local and intrathoracic extension of thyroid goitre or carcinoma;
- detect cervical or thoracic metastatic disease.

Postcontrast CT (Fig. 3.15) was performed in this patient and demonstrates an irregular, low-attenuation mass in the right lobe of the thyroid (black arrow) which invades the trachea (small white arrow). The normal left lobe is demonstrated (curved arrow).

Further reading

Hussain, H., Britton, K. & Grossman, A. (1998) Thyroid cancer. In: *Imaging in Oncology* (eds J.E. Husband & R.H. Resnek), 1st edn, pp. 481–514. Isis Medical Media Ltd, Oxford.

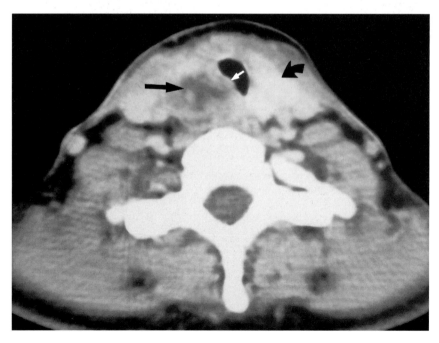

Fig. 3.15

CASE 8

A 60-year-old female presents with right upper quadrant discomfort and increasing abdominal distension. No abdominal mass is palpable.

What does the supine abdominal radiograph (Fig. 3.16) demonstrate?
What causes should be considered?
What further investigations are indicated?

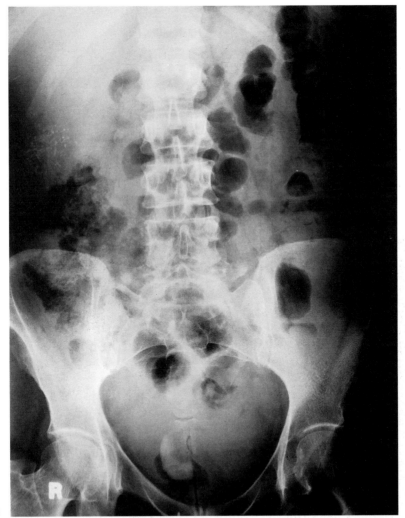

Fig. 3.16

The abdominal radiograph (Fig. 3.16) demonstrates amorphous, stippled calcifications in the right upper quadrant in the right lobe of the liver, lateral to the kidney. A further cluster of calcifications can be seen to the right of the lower lumbar spine.

The multiplicity and configuration of these calcifications are highly suspicious for metastatic mucinous adenocarcinoma involving the liver and para-aortic nodes. Primary sites include rectum, colon, ovary or stomach.

Postcontrast CT imaging (Fig. 3.17) confirmed a low-attenuation mass in the right lobe of the liver containing multiple calcifications (black arrow). There are enlarged para-aortic nodes also (curved black arrows). Ascites is present (white arrow). Pelvic ultrasound demonstrated a normal postmenopausal uterus and ovaries. Percutaneous biopsy of the hepatic lesion, using CT guidance, confirmed metastatic mucin-secreting adenocarcinoma of large bowel origin.

Hepatic calcification

Hepatic calcification, seen on an abdominal radiograph in adults, may be due to the following.

Granulomata
Typically single or multiple, rounded calcifications. Often following tuberculosis infection.

Phleboliths
Rounded calcifications, often with central lucency.

Hydatid disease
Twenty to thirty per cent of hydatid cysts may calcify, often with an 'eggshell' appearance.

Old abscesses or haematomas
Calcification is often curvilinear.

Hepatoma
Punctate, stippled or granular calcifications.

Metastases
Punctate, stippled or granular. Calcification may occur in lesions post-radiotherapy or chemotherapy.

Further reading

Darlak, J.J., Moskowitz, M. & Katten, K.R. (1980) Calcifications within the liver. *Radiologic Clinics of North America* **18**, 209–219.

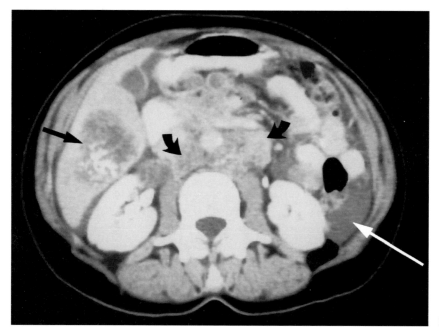

Fig. 3.17

CASE 9

A 26-year-old male presents with increasing shortness of breath and mild epigastric discomfort following a motorcycle accident.

What does the erect chest radiograph (Fig. 3.18) demonstrate?
What diagnosis should be considered?
What further investigations may help management?

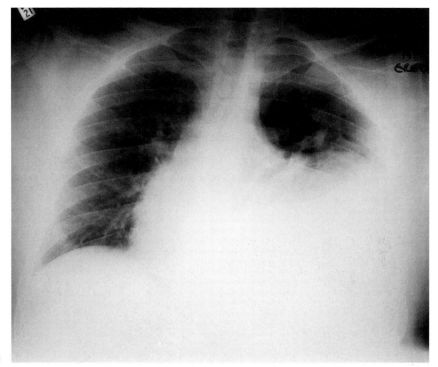

Fig. 3.18

The chest radiograph (Fig. 3.18) demonstrates a focus of linear atelectasis in the left mid-zone with pronounced elevation of the left hemidiaphragm. The left heart border is not well visualized but there is evidence of tracheal and right heart border deviation to the right. The radiographic appearances are suspicious for traumatic rupture of the left diaphragm.

Postcontrast CT imaging of the chest and abdomen (Fig. 3.19) confirmed the left chest to be filled with mesenteric fat and bowel loops (arrow) and the spleen was also abnormally rotated and intrathoracic (curved arrow).

Traumatic diaphragmatic hernia

- Results from blunt or penetrating trauma.
- Presentation may be delayed for months or years following initial trauma.
- Commonly left-sided (stomach, colon and small bowel most often involved).
- Life-threatening strangulation of contents is a serious hazard.

- Associated injuries include lower rib fractures, viscus perforation and splenic rupture.

The chest radiograph is the most useful initial investigation in diagnosing acute diaphragmatic rupture, although serial radiographs may be needed. An abnormally positioned nasogastric tube may be evident. Barium studies may also be helpful.

CT imaging is highly specific in making the diagnosis. Coronal reconstruction of the axial images may help in visualization of the extent of the diaphragmatic defect and assessment of the associated soft tissue and bony injuries.

Further reading

Murray, J.G., Caoili, E., Gruden, J.F., Evans, S.J., Halvorsen, R.A. & Mackersie, R.C. (1996) Acute rupture of the diaphragm due to blunt trauma: diagnostic sensitivity and specificity of computed tomography. *American Journal of Roentgenology* **166**, 1035–1039.

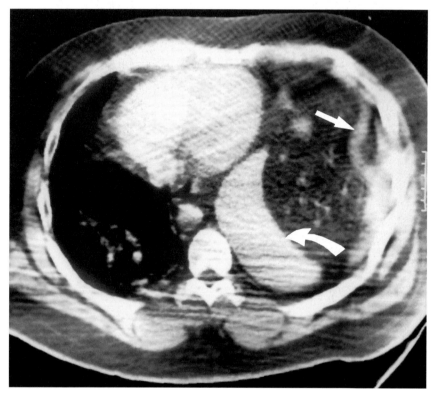

Fig. 3.19

CASE 10

A 20-year-old male presents with acute pain on swallowing (odynophagia) following a meal.

What does the lateral cervical spine radiograph (Fig. 3.20) show?

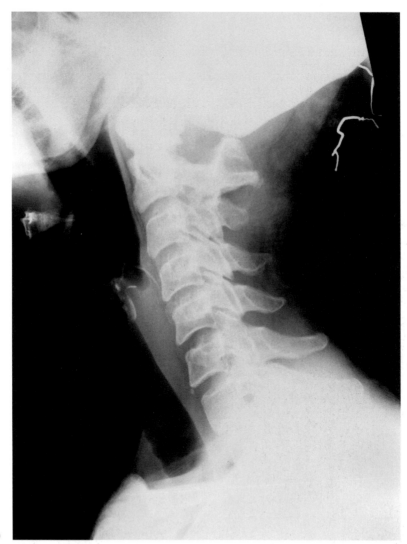

Fig. 3.20

On the reproduced lateral radiograph of the neck (Fig. 3.21) there is evidence of a curvilinear impacted bone at the level of the pyriform fossae (curved arrow) with air in the prevertebral soft tissues (small arrows).

Many sorts of foreign bodies are swallowed, whether accidentally or intentionally, by children and adults alike. Metallic objects are usually obvious on plain radiography. Pieces of bone lodge most commonly in the cervical oesophagus.

Plain radiographs

Pitfalls of plain radiographs in identifying objects impacted in the oesophagus:
• The degree and nature of normal laryngeal cartilage ossification.
• The type of bone ingested. Meat and chicken bones tend to be relatively radiodense and visible on radiographs, with many fish bones relatively radiolucent.

When no abnormality is seen on plain radiograph a barium swallow, with or without bolus, may help demonstrate the presence of an impacted foreign body.

Perforation of the oesophageal wall can cause air to enter prevertebral soft tissue, as in this case. If the foreign body is retained for some time sepsis may occur, with soft tissue swelling and air demonstrable in pharyngeal soft tissues.

Endoscopic examination may visualize an impacted foreign body and then allow removal. It is advisable to remove sharp or toxic objects to avoid the risk of perforation or caustic erosion. Blunt and non-toxic objects can be allowed to pass normally spontaneously, provided the patient is asymptomatic. In some instances dormier basket extraction can be performed under fluoroscopic control.

Further reading

Simpkins, K.C. (1993) The salivary glands, pharynx and oesophagus. In: *A Textbook of Radiology and Imaging* (ed. D. Sutton), 5th edn, pp. 783–786. Churchill Livingstone, Edinburgh.

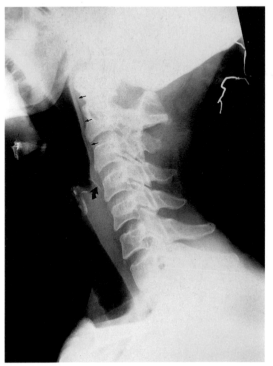

Fig. 3.21

CASE 11

A 70-year-old male presents with progressive abdominal pain and accompanying pyrexia. An abdominal mass is palpable in the right upper quadrant.

What is the most striking feature on the supine abdominal radiograph (Fig. 3.22)?
How can this be confirmed?
What other diagnosis should be considered?

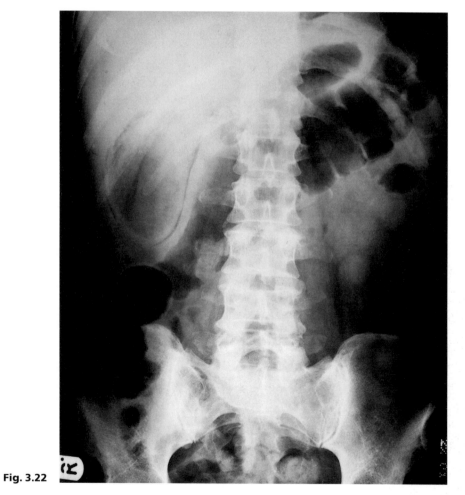

Fig. 3.22

In the right upper quadrant of the abdominal radiograph (Fig. 3.22) there is a thick-walled viscus with air identified in its wall. The configuration and position of the abnormality suggest that it is an abnormal gall bladder and the air in the wall is consistent with the diagnosis of emphysematous cholecystitis.

Ultrasound, the initial investigation of choice (Fig. 3.23), confirmed a distended gall bladder (large white arrow) containing hypoechoic bile and more echogenic sludge posteriorly (curved open arrows). The posterior wall of the gall bladder is hyperechoic, consistent with air in the wall (small white arrows). No calculi were seen.

Emphysematous cholecystitis

Due to calculus (70–80%) or acalculus cystic duct obstruction with inflammatory oedema and resultant cystic artery occlusion. Secondary infection supervenes, commonly with *Escherichia coli* or gas-forming organisms such as *Clostridium perfringens*.

- The condition is more common in elderly males.
- Diabetics and those with chronic, debilitating diseases are predisposed.
- Inflammatory indices may be normal.
- Complications include gallbladder gangrene and perforation.
- Mortality is high.

Ultrasound and CT imaging both help delineate the gall bladder further and can demonstrate air in the thickened gallbladder wall. Both modalities will visualize associated biliary tree dilatation, obstructing calculus or fluid collections, and will allow differentiation from an air-containing abscess in relation to perforated duodenum or malpositioned appendix, which may cause similar radiographic appearances.

Further reading

Laing, F.C. (1992) Ultrasonography of the acute abdomen. *Radiologic Clinics of North America* **30**, 389–404.

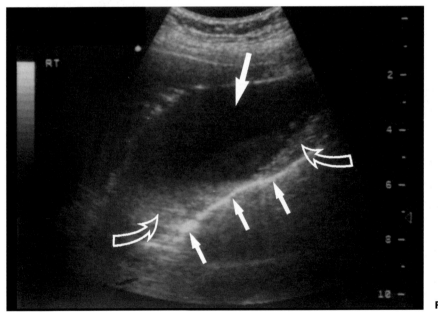

Fig. 3.23

CASE 12

A 45-year-old female presents with a 1-year history of a slowly enlarging, painless swelling in her right parotid gland. Ultrasound was performed (Fig. 3.24).

What normal structure is highlighted by arrows (Fig. 3.24)?
What abnormality is demonstrated and what is the likely diagnosis?
What further imaging may be helpful in further assessment?

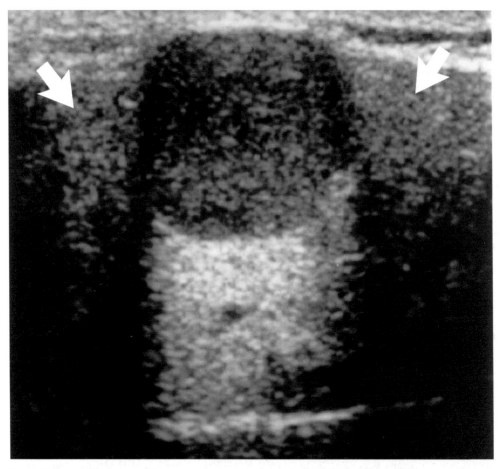

Fig. 3.24

The arrows (Fig. 3.24) indicate normal parotid tissue. However, centrally and within the superficial lobe of the right parotid gland is a well-circumscribed, hypoechoic and solid mass with associated distal acoustic enhancement. These ultrasound appearances are consistent with a benign parotid tumour likely to represent a pleomorphic adenoma. Ultrasound-guided biopsy confirmed this diagnosis and superficial parotidectomy was performed.

Benign parotid tumours

- Pleomorphic adenoma
- Cystadenolymphoma (Warthin's tumour) often multifocal and internal cystic changes are common.
- Oncocytoma: 1% of lesions.
- Haemangioma: more common in children.
- Lipoma.
- Neurogenic tumour.

Ultrasound is the most useful investigation for initial assessment of palpable parotid abnormalities, though caveats exist.

Most salivary gland tumours occur in the parotid gland and 80% of these are pleomorphic adenomas. These usually present as slowly growing, asymptomatic masses in young or middle-aged patients. On ultrasound pleomorphic adenomas usually appear well circumscribed and of homogeneous echotexture, with no related adenopathy. Ultrasound cannot visualize the facial nerve, and the deep lobe of the parotid gland may be obscured by overlying

bone. Ultrasound will demonstrate the intraparotid external carotid artery and retromandibular vein, however, and can demonstrate lesions superficial to these to be confined to the superficial aspect of the gland. Ultrasound-guided biopsy or fine-needle aspiration can also be performed if required.

For assessment of the deep lobe of the parotid gland and parotid malignancy, MR is the imaging modality of choice. MR imaging is able to differentiate between both the intraparotid vessels and the intraparotid portion of the facial nerve, and due to its multiplanar capacity is able to delineate deep extension of parotid neoplasms. Pleomorphic adenomas usually appear as high signal on MR T2-weighted images due to their high myxoid content and they tend to enhance homogeneously following gadolinium administration.

An axial T2-weighted MR image (Fig. 3.25) in a different patient presenting with dysphagia shows a large, well-circumscribed mass of relatively homogeneous high signal (arrow) arising from the deep lobe of the right parotid gland (curved arrow), with extension into the parapharyngeal space. Subsequent histology confirmed a pleomorphic adenoma.

Further reading

Soler, R., Bargiela, A., Requejo, I., Rodriguez, E., Rey, J.L. & Sancristan, F. (1997) Pictorial review: MR imaging of parotid tumours. *Clinical Radiology* **52**, 269–275.

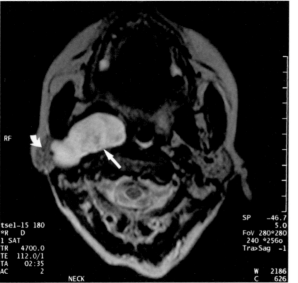

Fig. 3.25

CHAPTER 4

David V. Hughes

CASE 1

A 40-year-old male involved in a high-speed road traffic accident complained of pain in the upper neck. No neurological abnormality was demonstrated on clinical examination.

What abnormality is demonstrated on the lateral radiograph (Fig. 4.1) of the upper cervical spine?
What further imaging is recommended?

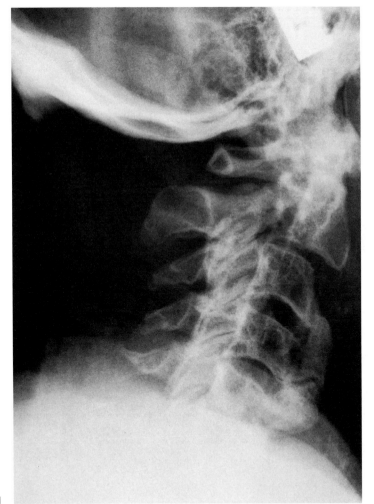

Fig. 4.1

The lateral cervical spine radiograph (Fig. 4.1) reveals a lucency seen through the pedicular region of the axis (C2) and subluxation of the axis anteriorly in relation to the C3 vertebral body. The features described are of a bilateral fracture through the neural arch of the axis. This is a traumatic spondylolisthesis or 'hangman's' fracture.

Classification of traumatic spondylolisthesis

• Type 1. No disruption of C2/3 disc with consequent normal alignment of C2/3 on the lateral radiograph.
• Type 2. Disruption of C2/3 disc allowing forward slip of C2 on C3.
• Type 3. Disruption of C2/3 disc with bilateral dislocation of interarticular facets of C2/3.

A bilateral pars interarticularis fracture of the axis is unstable. This injury, which may follow a high-speed road traffic accident, results from forceful hyperextension of the cervical spine. The term 'hangman's' fracture derives from the similar traumatic features found in those executed by judicial hanging.

Confirmation and more accurate delineation of cervical spine fractures can be achieved by CT imaging. In this patient the CT image (Fig. 4.2) demonstrates the C2 neural arch fractures (arrows) with adjacent extensive haematoma posteriorly (open arrows). There is also a fracture of the right intervertebral foramen (curved arrow).

For spinal fractures CT imaging will provide good definition of bony architecture, which is particularly useful when it is suspected that bony fragments have been displaced into the spinal canal. However, accurate assessment of underlying spinal cord injury is best assessed by MR imaging.

Further reading

Harris, J.H., Harris, W.H. & Novelline, R.A. (1993) Spine including soft tissues of phorynx & neck. In: *The Radiology of Emergency Medicine*, 3rd edn, pp. 127–282. Williams & Wilkins, Baltimore.
Effendi, B., Roy, D., Cornish, B. *et al.* (1981) Fractures of the ring of the axis: a classification based on the analysis of 131 cases. *Journal of Bone and Joint Surgery* **63B**, 319–327.

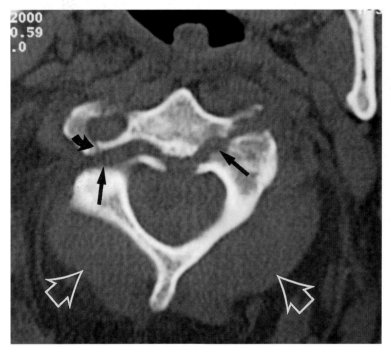

Fig. 4.2

CASE 2

A 59-year-old male presents with a history of urinary frequency. No organisms are demonstrated on urinary culture for suspected urinary tract infection.

What is the abnormality demonstrated on supine abdominal radiograph (Fig. 4.3)?
Is a chest radiograph pertinent?
What further radiological investigations are recommended?

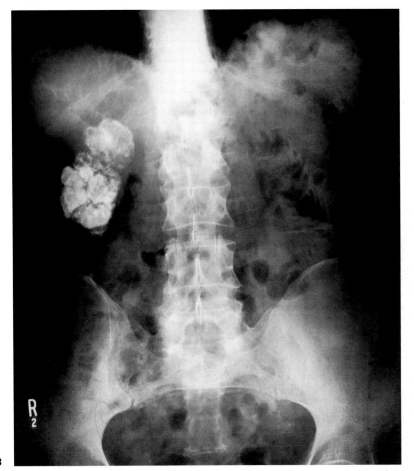

Fig. 4.3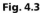

The abdominal radiograph (Fig. 4.3) reveals a small scarred right kidney with diffuse dystrophic calcification distributed in a lobular configuration throughout. The appearances are consistent with late-stage renal tuberculosis and autonephrectomy.

Urinary tract tuberculosis

• Second most common site after respiratory tract.
• Adult males affected more frequently than females (ratio 3 : 1).
• Associated with sterile pyuria.
• Many will have a history of previous tuberculous infection, usually pulmonary.

A chest radiograph may reveal evidence of previous or current tuberculosis in as many as 50% of patients.

An intravenous urogram (Fig. 4.4), from another patient, demonstrates many of the urinary tract manifestations of tuberculosis. There is a stricture at the left vesico-ureteric junction with hydronephrosis and hydroureter proximally. The bladder is shrunken and there is contrast leakage via a fistula (arrow) into a perivesical collection. This patient also has a right autonephrectomy partially obscured by bowel gas.

CT imaging can provide further information on morphological abnormalities such as scarring, calcification, hydronephrosis and extrarenal disease.

Further reading

Leder, R.A. & Low, V.H.S. (1995) Tuberculosis of the abdomen. *Radiologic Clinics of North America* **33**, 691–705.

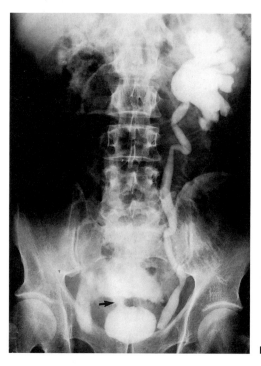

Fig. 4.4

CASE 3

A 50-year-old female with a history of carcinoma of the cervix presents with left-sided abdominal discomfort.

What abnormal findings are there on the radiograph (Fig. 4.5) taken during an intravenous urogram series?
What further investigation would you request?

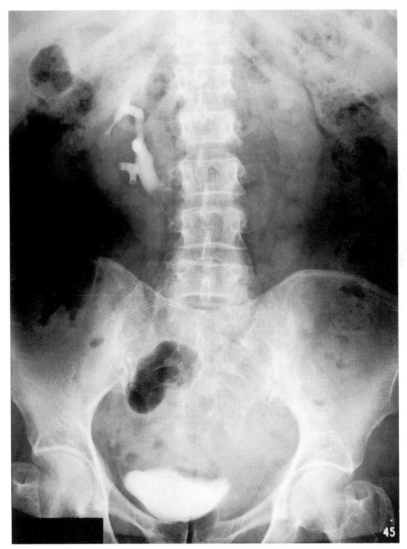

Fig. 4.5

The radiograph from the intravenous urogram series (Fig. 4.5) shows the long axes of the nephrograms to be vertically orientated with an isthmus of renal tissue bridging the lower poles of the kidneys (horseshoe kidney). There is no urogram on the left, indicative of obstruction on this side. There is a soft tissue mass in the left pelvis displacing the bladder to the right and there is erosion of the mucosa of the left bladder, raising the suspicion of extrinsic invasion by a local mass.

Horseshoe kidney

• Most common renal fusion abnormality.
• Usually it is the lower poles that are joined by renal tissue or a fibrous band.

• The fused segment lies below the inferior mesenteric artery, preventing full renal ascent.
• The more ventral ureteric positions predispose to obstruction by crossing aberrant vessels.

The postcontrast CT image (Fig. 4.6) demonstrates the isthmus of the horseshoe kidney (open arrow) with the left moiety hydronephrotic. The more caudal CT image (Fig. 4.7), on the same patient, confirms the presence of a large, irregular mass in the left pelvis displacing and invading the bladder wall on the left side (arrows). These features are consistent with this patient's locally advanced cervical cancer.

Further reading

Platt, J.F. (1996) Urinary obstruction. *Radiologic Clinics of North America* **34**, 1113–1129.

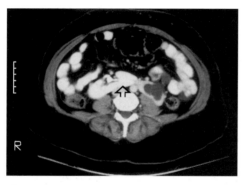

Fig. 4.6

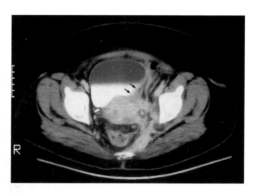

Fig. 4.7

CASE 4

A 22-year-old male presents with a hard, painless swelling in the right scrotum. Initially scrotal ultrasound was performed.

What do the longitudinal images of the right (Fig. 4.8) and left (Fig. 4.9) testes demonstrate?
What is the diagnosis?

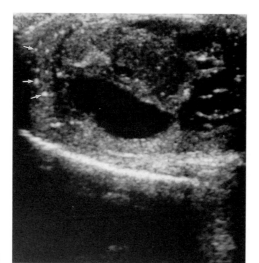

Fig. 4.8

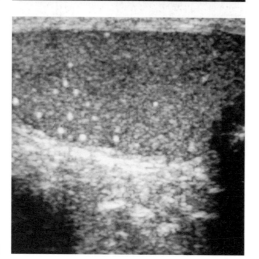

Fig. 4.9

There is a large complex solid and cystic mass replacing most of the right testis (Fig. 4.8). The left testis (Fig. 4.9) contains scattered internal foci of calcification and some microcalcifications can also be seen at the upper pole of the right testis (small arrows).

This patient has bilateral testicular microlithiasis and a complicating teratoma (confirmed at surgery) of the right testis.

Testicular microlithiasis (TM)

• Due to calcium deposits in the lumina of the seminiferous tubules.
• Increasingly recognized with ultrasound.
• The calcifications have characteristic ultrasound appearances and appear as speckled, echogenic foci.

• Aetiology is unclear although may be post-inflammatory.

It is now appreciated that there is an association between TM and germ-cell neoplasia. Seminoma is the tumour most frequently observed, although teratomas do occur (as in this case).

All patients with TM should have regular clinical follow-up with accompanying tumour marker estimation and testicular ultrasound.

Testicular ultrasound in another patient (Fig. 4.10) demonstrates an atrophic testis containing florid microlithiasis.

Further reading

Howlett, D.C., Marchbank, N.D. & Sallomi, D.F. (2000) Ultrasound of the testis. *Clinical Radiology* **55**, 595–601.

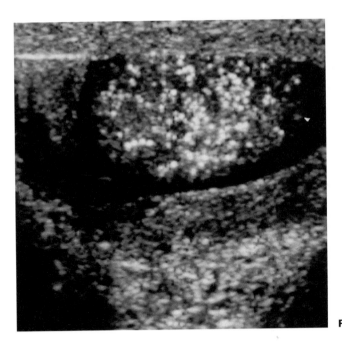

Fig. 4.10

CASE 5

An 11-month-old infant is being investigated for recurrent urinary tract infection.

What is this investigation (Fig. 4.11)?
What are the abnormal radiological findings?

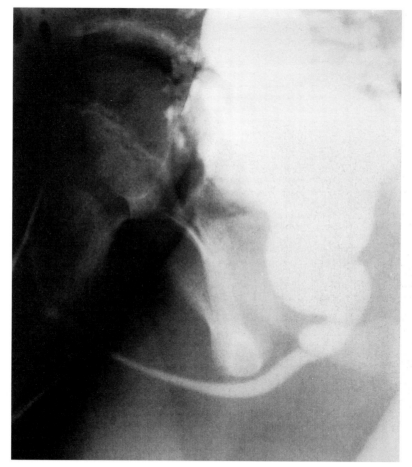

Fig. 4.11

The reproduced radiograph (Fig. 4.12) is of the bladder taken during a micturating cystogram. The abnormalities shown include:

- hypertrophied, trabeculated, sacculated bladder (open arrows);
- dilatation of posterior urethra (curved arrow);
- posterior urethral valve (small arrow).

The features result from posterior urethral valves. These are thickened folds of mucosa found within the posterior urethra distal to the verumontanum. Additional changes observed, in this condition, during a micturating cystogram include vesico-ureteric reflux, usually left-sided, and a large postmicturition residual urine.

Bladder outflow obstruction

Causes of bladder outflow obstruction in a male child:

- Posterior urethral valves.
- Vesical or urethral diverticulum.
- Urethral stricture.
- Calculus.
- Prune belly syndrome.
- Meatal stenosis.
- Phimosis.

Further reading

Auni, E.F., Dicks-Mireaux, C., Neuenschwander, S. & Van Gansbeke, D. (1994) The urinary tract. In: *Imaging Children*, Vol. 1 (eds H. Carty, N. Shaw, F. Brunelle & B. Kendall), pp. 561–754. Churchill Livingstone, London.

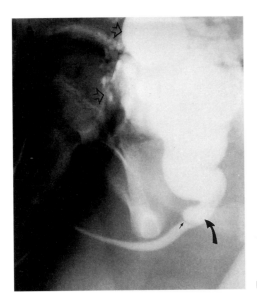

Fig. 4.12

CASE 6

A 73-year-old male presents with weight loss and haematuria.

From what study is this radiograph (Fig. 4.13) taken?
What is the most likely diagnosis?
What alternative imaging techniques can provide additional useful information?

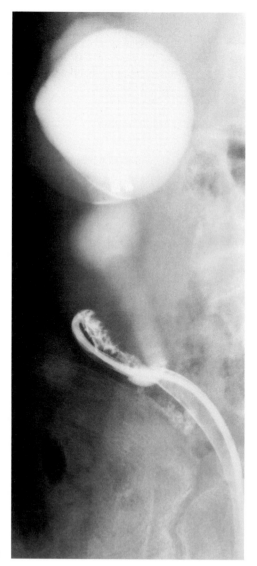

Fig. 4.13

The radiograph (Fig. 4.13) is taken during a right retrograde ureterogram in which the passage of the ureteric catheter to the renal pelvis has been prevented by an irregular shouldered stricture within the mid-ureter. Proximal obstruction is clearly evident. These appearances are due to ureteric transitional cell carcinoma (TCC). A further right retrograde study (Fig. 4.14) from another patient shows more extensive TCC involvement of the upper tract with changes throughout the upper ureter and renal pelvis (arrows).

Ureteric TCC

- Male predominance.
- Peak incidence in seventh decade.
- Lower third of ureter is the most common site.
- Synchronous and metachronous lesions are common.
- Predisposing factors include: bladder TCC, analgesic nephropathy, aniline dye/cyclophosphamide/tobacco exposure.

Imaging features of TCC

Plain radiograph
Coarse punctuate calcification may be present.

Intravenous urogram
Pelvicalyceal and upper ureteric filling defects, non-functioning kidney.

Retrograde ureterogram
Filling defects/strictures.

Ultrasound scan
Pelvicalyceal dilatation/hypoechoic mass. Mass lesions in bladder.

CT imaging
Used to stage the disease and determine resectability by revealing local extent of tumour and evidence of nodal or more distant spread.

Further reading

Winalski, C.S., Lipman, J.C. & Tumeh, S.S. (1990) Ureteral neoplasms. *Radiographics* **10**, 271–283.

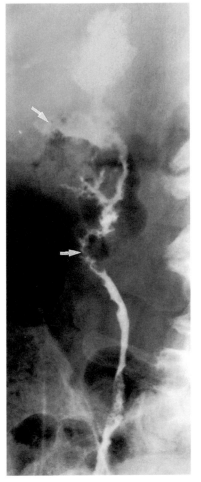

Fig. 4.14

CASE 7

A 78-year-old male presents with rapid weight loss and epigastric discomfort.

What radiographic abnormality is shown on the radiograph from a barium meal series (Fig. 4.15)?
What possible pathological entities may give rise to this appearance?
What additional radiological investigations may be helpful?

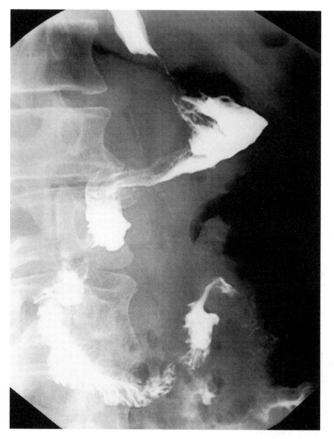

Fig. 4.15

The radiograph from a barium meal series (Fig. 4.15) reveals a narrowed non-distensible body and antrum of stomach with destruction of the normal mucosal pattern. There is mucosal abnormality also within the fundus, extending into the lower oesophagus which is strictured. Loss of peristalsis in the abnormal segment could be appreciated on fluoroscopic inspection at the time of the examination. The differential diagnosis includes advanced carcinoma of the stomach (linitis plastica), metastatic infiltration (commonly by carcinoma of the breast) or lymphoma. An upper gastrointestinal endoscopy with biopsies confirmed a diagnosis of a diffusely infiltrated carcinoma of the stomach in this patient.

Linitis plastica (leather-bottle) gastric carcinoma

- Characterized by extensive infiltration of the submucosa and muscular layers.
- Marked fibroblastic/desmoplastic reaction around the columns of malignant cells.
- Endoscopic recognition may be difficult and superficial biopsies negative.
- Prognosis is poor.

Radiological staging of gastric carcinoma

CT imaging
This is the mainstay for staging purposes, allowing assessment of tumour size, adjacent visceral involvement, lymph node enlargement and metastatic spread (liver, adrenals, ovaries, bone, peritoneal seeding and ascites).

In the patient's postcontrast CT image from another patient with gastric carcinoma (Fig. 4.16), multiple low-attenuation lesions are seen throughout the liver indicating widespread hepatic metastases.

Endoscopic ultrasound
This can provide increased accuracy in the demonstration of depth of tumour invasion and will also yield useful information on invasion of local structures and lymph node enlargement.

Further reading

Miller, F.H., Kochman, M.L., Talamonti, M.S., Ghahremani, G.G. & Gore R.M. (1997) Gastric cancer (radiologic staging). *Radiologic Clinics of North America* **35**, 331–349.

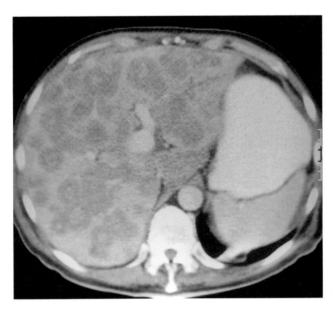

Fig. 4.16

CASE 8

A 25-year-old male who has fallen on his outstretched hand presents with a painful, swollen right wrist.

What abnormality is shown on the anteroposterior (AP) and lateral radiographs of the right wrist (Fig. 4.17)?
What carpal bone is arrowed?

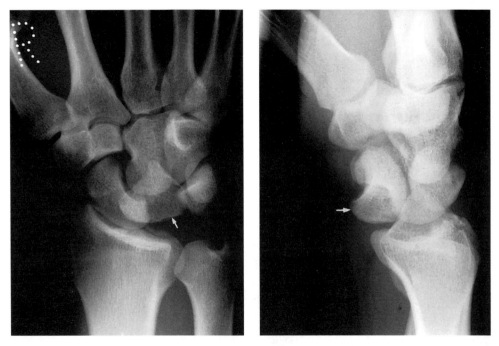

Fig. 4.17

These radiographs (Fig. 4.17) demonstrate a lunate dislocation (stage IV carpal instability). On the AP view the lunate (arrowed) assumes a triangular shape with consequent loss of its normal relationship with adjacent carpals. The lateral view shows the lunate to be displaced anteriorly and rotated through 90°, such that its convex surface is dorsal. This injury represents disruption of several joints and ligaments, leading to instability of the carpus of the most severe form.

Carpal instability

Classification of carpal instability (in order of increasing severity).
• Stage I. Isolated rotatory subluxation of the scaphoid. On an AP radiograph this is seen as widening of the scapholunate space ('Terry Thomas' sign).
• Stage II. The radiographic features are demonstrated on the AP (Fig. 4.18) and lateral (Fig. 4.19) views of a right wrist. There is disruption of the capitate–lunate joint with resultant

posterior dislocation of the carpal bones (Fig. 4.19, open arrows). Radiolunate alignment is theoretically maintained, although some lunate rotation invariably occurs, creating its triangular appearance on the AP radiograph (Fig. 4.18). This view also shows a trans-scaphoid fracture (curved arrow) and furthermore a triquetral fracture (straight arrow).
• Stage III. As for Stage II but with triquetral dislocation and a greater degree of ligamentous disruption.
• Stage IV. The lunate rotates approximately 90° in the volar direction. A lateral radiograph establishes the diagnosis and shows that the capitate occupies the space left by the lunate. This injury is also commonly associated with trans-scaphoid fracture.

Further reading

Harris, J.H., Jr, Harris, W.H. & Novelline, R.A. (1993) Wrist. In: *The Radiology of Emergency Medicine*, 3rd edn, pp. 375–434. Williams & Wilkins, Baltimore.

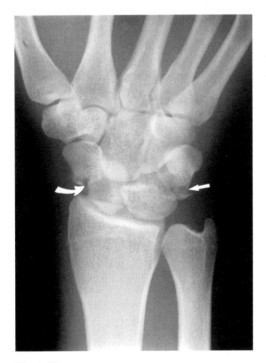

Fig. 4.18

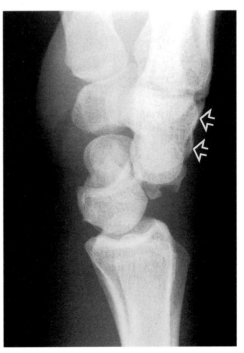

Fig. 4.19

CASE 9

A 55-year-old man hit his head on concrete when falling from a ladder. Anteroposterior (Fig. 4.20) and lateral (Fig. 4.21) skull radiographs are shown.

What abnormalities are demonstrated?
What do the arrows highlight?

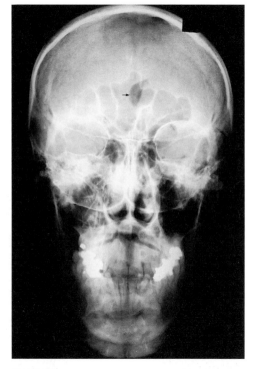

Fig. 4.20

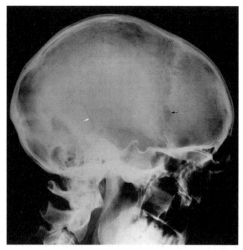

Fig. 4.21

The lateral skull radiograph (Fig. 4.21) demonstrates a linear, well-defined lucency projecting over the parietal bone, indicating an acute fracture at this site (white arrow). Additionally, there is lucency seen on both radiographic views (Figs 4.20 & 4.21) within the skull vault, in the position of and conforming to the shape of the anterior horn of the left lateral ventricle (black arrows). This represents intraventricular air secondary to the fracture.

Causes of intracranial air

- Trauma.
- Neoplasm.
- Infection with a gas-forming organism.
- Post-surgery.

Following trauma, intracranial air is indicative of the compound nature of a fracture. Fractures extending to involve paranasal sinuses (frontal, ethmoid and sphenoid) with breach of a dura mater are commonly implicated. Intracranial air is rarely evident at presentation and may accumulate over days, weeks or even months. Follow-up skull radiographs of fractures involving the sinuses (the lateral brow-up position with horizontal beam) should therefore be performed where there is clinical concern or cerebrospinal fluid rhinorrhoea, or otorrhoea persists. The unenhanced CT image through the basal cisterns of the brain in another patient (Fig. 4.22) demonstrates the presence of post-traumatic subarachnoid air (arrows).

Further reading

Sutton, D. (1993) The skull. In: *A Textbook of Radiology and Imaging*, 5th edn, pp. 1377–1406. Churchill Livingstone, Edinburgh.

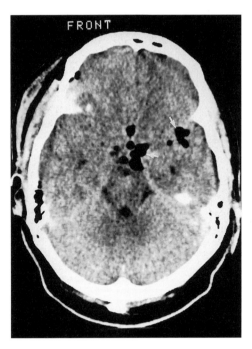

Fig. 4.22

CASE 10

A 64-year-old female presents with bowel disturbance and rectal bleeding. Rigid sigmoidoscopy identifies a polypoid lesion at the rectosigmoid junction.

What abnormality is shown on the lateral radiograph of the rectosigmoid region (Fig. 4.23) taken during a barium enema examination?

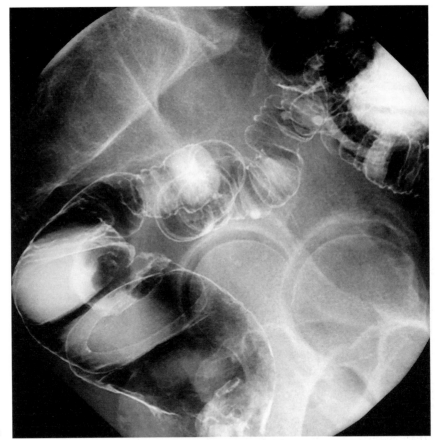

Fig. 4.23

There is a 3-cm polypoidal filling defect seen on the anterior wall at the rectosigmoid junction on this lateral view (Fig. 4.23) from a double-contrast barium enema. The anterior mucosa is puckered and irregular. Biopsy confirmed malignant change in an adenomatous polyp.

Malignant transformation of a polyp: key barium enema features

• Broad irregular base.
• Large polyp (greater than 2 cm diameter) with associated mucosal irregularity.
• Progressive growth on sequential studies.
• 'Soap bubble' surface indicative of villous content (which is a risk factor for malignant change).

Double-contrast barium enema versus colonoscopy

Much debate surrounds the best method of diagnosing polyps. A good quality double-contrast barium enema can reliably detect polyps 0.5 cm or more in diameter. Smaller polyps may be seen on colonoscopy with the added advantage of allowing simultaneous treatment. With barium enema there is a higher chance of technical suc-cess in examining the entire colon and it may demonstrate lesions behind mucosal folds not visible to the endoscopist. Colonoscopy may represent the investigation of choice in the presence of a tortuous sigmoid colon which contains multiple diverticula, where resolution of a polyp radiologically is often difficult. When a polyp is suspected clinically, colonoscopy is the preferred imaging technique and this modality will also identify flat lesions occult radiologically. Complications of colonoscopy include perforation and haemorrhage, although these are rare.

Alternative imaging techniques for large rectal polyps/cancers include CT imaging with or without pneumocolon, endo-anal ultrasound and MR imaging with or without an intracavitary coil. Figure 4.24 is an axial image through the rectum from a CT pneumocolon examination. In this technique postcontrast CT imaging is combined with an intravenous antispasmodic agent and rectal air insufflation. A plaque-like rectal carcinoma, with central ulceration (arrow), is well demonstrated within the air-filled rectum.

Further reading

Smith, C. (1997) Colorectal cancer (radiologic diagnosis). *Radiologic Clinics of North America* **35**, 439–456.

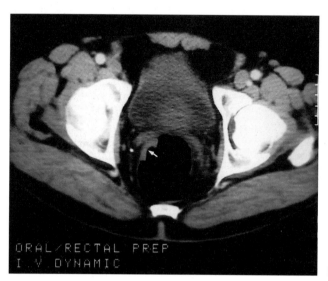
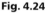

Fig. 4.24

CASE 11

A 34-year-old male presents with enlarged inguinal and axillary lymph nodes, weight loss and diarrhoea.

What abnormality is shown on the radiograph (Fig. 4.25) taken from a small bowel barium study?
What differential diagnosis is there for this appearance?

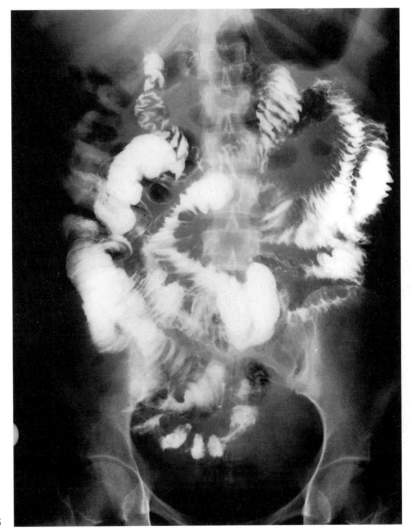

Fig. 4.25

The radiograph (Fig. 4.25) from the small bowel barium study shows diffuse, irregular thickening of mucosal folds throughout the small bowel. Moreover the bowel loops appear to be separated due to mural thickening. Endoscopy and biopsy confirmed diffuse infiltration with T-cell lymphoma.

Mucosal fold thickening

Causes of mucosal fold thickening in non-dilated small bowel (defined as greater than 2.5 mm in the jejunum and greater than 2 mm in the ileum).

Smooth regular folds
• Coeliac disease: uncommon (and should raise the possibility of complicating lymphoma).
• Oedema: hypoproteinaemic, angioneurotic, lymphatic.

• Vascular: haematoma secondary to trauma or bleeding diathesis; ischaemia due to embolus or vasculitis.
• Amyloidosis.
• Radiation.

Irregular and distorted folds
• Inflammatory: Crohn's disease.
• Infestation: giardiasis.
• Neoplastic: lymphoma, carcinoid or metastases.
   Marked mural thickening of the third part of the duodenum and proximal jejunum can be readily appreciated in the postcontrast CT image (Fig. 4.26) performed to stage this patient's disease.

Further reading

Herlinger, H., Maglinte, D.D.T., Birndaum, B.B. (1999) *Clinical Radiology of the Small Intestine.* Springer-Verlag, New York.

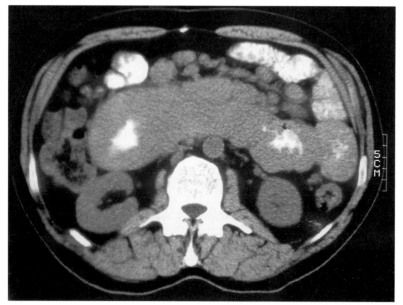

Fig. 4.26

CASE 12

An 84-year-old female with long-standing lower abdominal discomfort and irregular bowel habit now presents with offensive vaginal discharge.

What abnormalities are shown on the oblique radiograph of the rectosigmoid region (Fig. 4.27) taken from her barium enema examination?

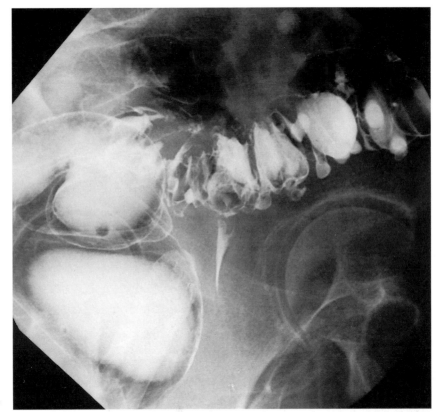

Fig. 4.27

The radiograph (Fig. 4.27) is reproduced below (Fig. 4.28). There is evidence of extensive sigmoid diverticular disease with associated circular muscle hypertrophy. Barium can be seen entering a fistulous track (Fig. 4.28, arrow) extending anteriorly and inferiorly towards the vagina.

Causes of colonic fistulae

• Inflammatory, e.g. Crohn's disease, diverticulitis, endometriosis.
• Neoplastic, e.g. carcinoma of the colon, cervix or vagina.
• Infection, e.g. tuberculosis, actinomycosis, lymphogranuloma venereum.
• Trauma/foreign body.
• Radiotherapy.

Diverticulosis is the commonest cause of colonic fistula formation, most frequently involving the bladder.

Radiological features of complications arising in diverticular disease

Plain radiograph
• Localized ileus or obstruction.
• Gas densities within abscess or fistula.

Barium enema
• Luminal narrowing by inflammatory mass.
• Thickening and distortion of mucosal folds.
• Pericolic sinus or collection.
• Fistula formation.

Further reading

Balthazar, E.J. (2000) Diverticular disease of the colon. In: *Textbook of Gastrointestinal Radiology* (eds R.M. Gore & M.S. Levine), 2nd edn, pp. 915–944. W.B. Saunders Co., Philadelphia.

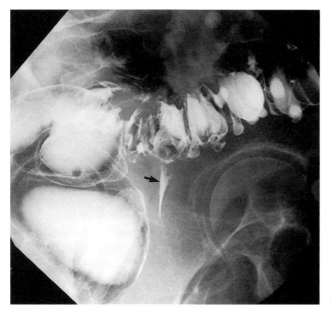

Fig. 4.28

CHAPTER 5

Nigel D.P. Marchbank

CASE 1

This 54-year-old man presented with a chronic history of bloody diarrhoea.

Abdominal and rectal examinations were unremarkable; however, rigid sigmoidoscopy revealed confluent mucosal ulceration with contact bleeding. A barium enema was requested.

What diagnosis can be made from the radiograph (Fig. 5.1) of this barium enema study?

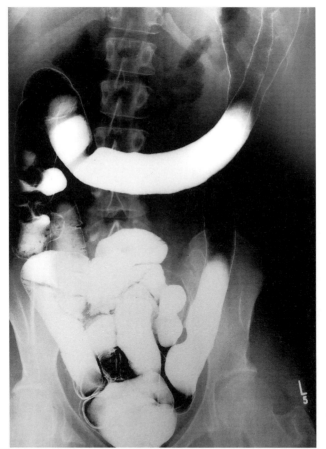

Fig. 5.1

The barium enema radiograph (Fig. 5.1) shows widespread, fine, mucosal ulceration of the distal colon and rectum giving rise to a rather granular appearance with loss of normal haustral pattern. The appearances are those of ulcerative colitis (UC).

Radiological features that favour a diagnosis of UC over Crohn's disease

• Granular mucosa rather than discrete aphthous ulceration or fissures.
• Rectal involvement.
• Disease in continuity.
• Haustral loss.

UC and Crohn's disease are the two most important forms of idiopathic inflammatory bowel disease. Distinction between the two is important and reflected in their clinicopathogenesis. UC invariably begins as a proctitis which may spread proximally to involve the whole colon.

The inflammatory changes are confined to the colonic and rectal mucosa only. Haemorrhage, toxic dilatation and perforation are acute complications. Malignant change may arise in extensive and long-standing (greater than 10 years' duration) UC. The radiograph (Fig. 5.2) from a barium enema series in another patient shows an irregular stricture with mucosal ulceration just distal to the splenic flexure (white arrows). This is a characteristic appearance of carcinoma in a patient with long-standing UC. There is also a small pseudopolyp in the transverse colon (curved white arrow).

Further reading

Gore, R.M., Laufer, I. & Berlin, J.W. (2000) Ulcerative and granulomatous Colitis. In: *Textbook of Gastrointestinal Radiology* (eds R.M. Gore & M.S. Levine), 2nd edn, pp. 945–992. W.B. Saunders Co., Philadelphia.

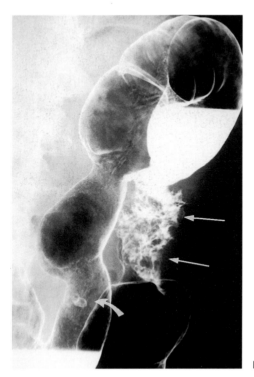

Fig. 5.2

CHAPTER 5

CASE 2

This 74-year-old woman developed right upper quadrant pain and fever 1 year following cholecystectomy. Abdominal ultrasound had shown no biliary dilatation or other abnormality.

What is this investigation (Fig. 5.3)?
What does it show?

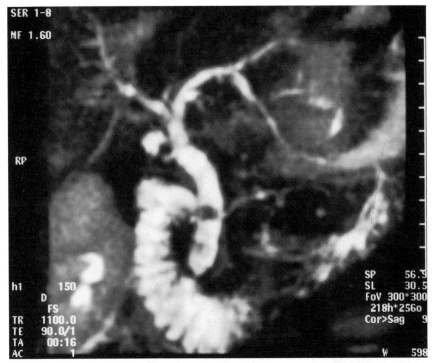

Fig. 5.3

Figures 5.3 and 5.4 (Fig. 5.3 reproduced) are images of an MR cholangiopancreatogram (MRCP). This patient has a patulous common bile duct with normal-calibre intrahepatic ducts. Two small filling defects within the lower portion of the common duct are due to calculi (black arrows). The main pancreatic duct (white arrow) and duodenal loop (white curved arrow) are also clearly seen.

Ultrasound remains the primary modality for the assessment of biliary disease. However, it is well recognized that small stones within a non-dilated biliary tree can be missed. MRCP, like ultrasound, is a non-invasive investigation of the pancreatic and biliary tree. MRCP is able to visualize the non-dilated common bile duct and can achieve a set of images that provide similar diagnostic information to endoscopic retrograde cholangiopancreatography (ERCP) and percutaneous transhepatic cholangiography (PTC).

Features of MR cholangiopancreatography

• Non-invasive investigation of pancreatic and biliary tree.
• Rapid acquisition during a single breath hold (the image reproduced in Fig. 5.4 took 16 s to acquire).
• Intravenous contrast agent not necessary.
• High diagnostic sensitivity.
• Safer and more economical diagnostic tool than ERCP and PTC.

Further reading

Hahn, P.F. (1999) Biliary System, pancreas, spleen and alimentary tract. In: *Magnetic Resonance Imaging* (eds D. Stark & W.G. Bradley Jr), pp. 471–499. Mosby Inc., St Louis, Missouri.

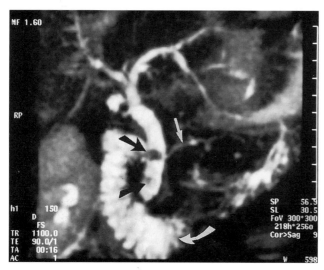

Fig. 5.4

CASE 3

This 84-year-old diabetic female presents with a 3-month history of crampy abdominal pains with diarrhoea. The pains were initially quite severe and associated with rectal bleeding. She had a normal barium enema 6 months previously.

What does this image from a repeat barium enema series (Fig. 5.5) show? What is the most likely diagnosis?

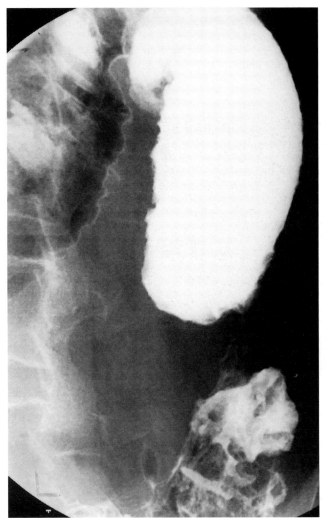

Fig. 5.5

The barium enema radiograph (Fig. 5.5) reveals a tight stricture in the descending colon. The mucosa within the stricture is reasonably smooth. There is marked mural oedema of the bowel on either side of the stricture with thumbprinting and thickening of the bowel wall.

The clinical history and radiological signs are strongly suggestive of ischaemic colitis.

Ischaemic colitis may present in an indolent fashion (as in this patient) or as an acute abdomen due to perforation with sepsis. The majority of patients are elderly with coexisting medical problems.

Outcomes of colonic ischaemia

- Stricture.
- Gangrene with secondary perforation.
- Persistent colitis.
- Spontaneous resolution and healing.

Where the presenting symptom of ischaemic colitis is abdominal pain and the plain radiograph is unhelpful, the patient is often initially investigated with ultrasound or CT imaging.

Non-specific changes of colitis, including symmetrical bowel thickening, polypoid defects associated with mural oedema and target or double halo pattern of the colon, may be observed. However, differentiation of an ischaemic cause from other forms of colitis can be made on the basis of sequential changes on barium enema.

Differential diagnosis of colonic strictures

- Malignant (carcinoma, lymphoma).
- Inflammatory (Crohn's disease, ulcerative colitis, radiotherapy, ischaemia).
- Infective (tuberculosis, amoebiasis, schistosomiasis, lymphogranuloma venereum).
- Extrinsic (tumours, inflammation, endometriosis).

Further reading

Toursarkissian, B. & Thompson, R.W. (1997) Ischaemic colitis. *Surgical Clinics of North America* **77**, 461–470.

CASE 4

This 56-year-old male developed sudden-onset, central, retrosternal chest pain.

What investigation has been undertaken (Fig. 5.6)?
What is the diagnosis?

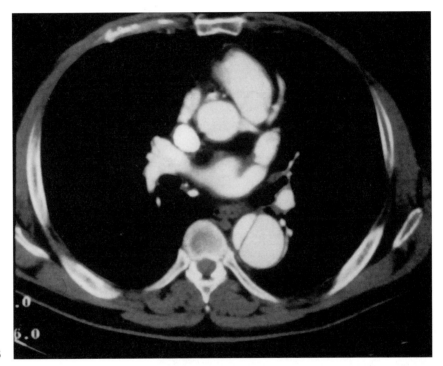

Fig. 5.6

This is a spiral, postcontrast CT image through the chest (Fig. 5.6). An intimal flap within the descending aorta is seen. In the sagittal reformat of the spiral acquisition (Fig. 5.7) in the same patient, the extent of the dissection is more apparent. Note that the true lumen (black arrow) and false lumen (white arrow) are clearly separated by the intimal flap (curved black arrow).

This patient has a type B aortic dissection (distal to the origin of the left subclavian artery). In type A dissection the dissection involves the aorta proximal to the left subclavian artery.

Aortic dissections occur as a result of disruption of both the intimal and medial layers.

Cystic medial necrosis and hypertension are important predisposing causes. Blood will collect within the aortic wall and either thrombose or create a false lumen when flowing blood communicates back again with the true lumen (Fig. 5.7).

Chest radiograph features of aortic dissection

- Widening and/or blurring of aortic shadow.
- Pleural effusion (usually on left).
- Tracheal shift.
- Displaced intimal calcification.

However, the chest radiograph may be entirely normal.

Spiral CT imaging and transoesophageal echocardiography have a high diagnostic sensitivity for aortic dissections. Indeed both are more accurate than formal angiography.

Further reading

Petasnic, J.P. (1991) Radiologic evaluation of aortic dissection. *Radiology* **180**, 297–305.

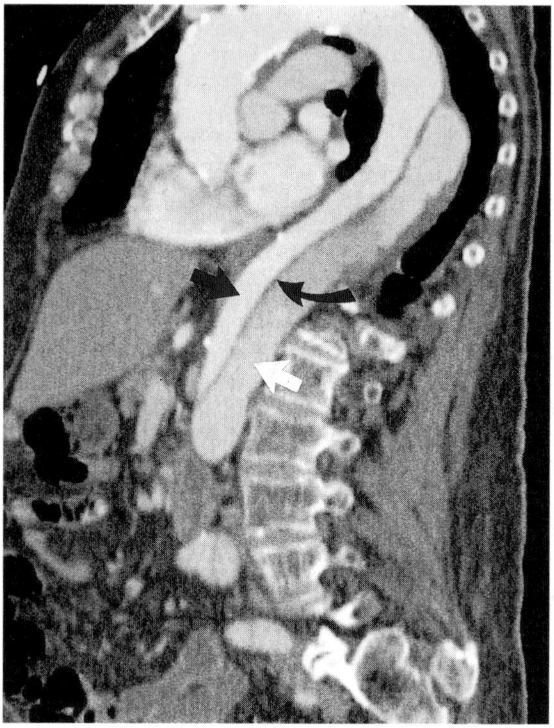

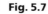

Fig. 5.7

CASE 5

This 32-year-old female, with a history of breast cancer, complains of severe low back pain. Lumbar radiographs were non-diagnostic.

What imaging technique is demonstrated (Fig. 5.8)?
What abnormalities are demonstrated?

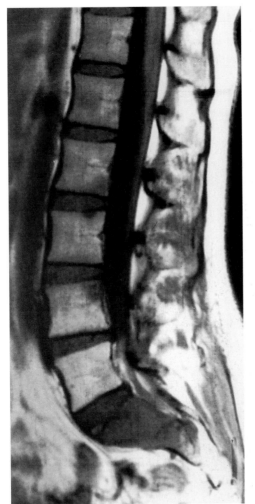

Fig. 5.8

A sagittal T1-weighted MR image of the lumbar spine is shown (Fig. 5.8).

The focused image (Fig. 5.9) highlights infiltration and destruction of the S1 vertebral body (black arrow). There is a further lesion within the posterior and superior aspect of the L4 vertebral body (white arrow).

This patient has radiological features of metastatic disease from carcinoma of the breast.

Imaging of suspected bony metastases

Radiographs

Widely available and commonly used as the first-line investigation. Metastases may be lytic, expansile lytic (renal and thyroid), sclerotic (breast and prostate) or mixed. Vertebral collapse associated with destruction of pedicles is strongly indicative of metastases. However, a collapsed vertebra alone may be due to trauma or osteoporosis. Radiographs are relatively insensitive and non-specific for metastatic disease.

Radionuclide imaging (bone scan)

High sensitivity for many metastatic tumours, particularly breast, lung and prostate. A typical positive test shows multiple asymmetrical areas of increased uptake. However, 5% of patients with bony metastases will have a normal scan. Moreover, specificity is poor since any area of increased bony activity will show as an area of increased isotope uptake.

MR imaging

High sensitivity in detecting marrow infiltration by metastases. Typically these are of low signal intensity on T1-weighted sequences (Fig. 5.9, white arrow). This modality can also be used to assess the extent of tumour spread outside the bone and is therefore of particular use within the spine for detecting cord compression.

Further reading

Söderlund, V. (1996) Radiological diagnosis of skeletal metastases. *European Radiology* **6**, 587–595.

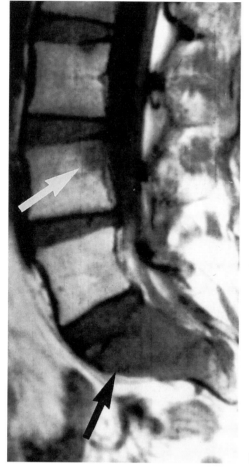

Fig. 5.9

CASE 6

This 26-year-old Asian male presented with a 3-month history of night sweats, weight loss and diarrhoea. Abdominal examination revealed a tender mass within the right iliac fossa. Digital rectal examination and rigid sigmoidoscopy were normal.

What is the radiological abnormality on this image from the barium enema examination (Fig. 5.10)?
What are the possible diagnoses?

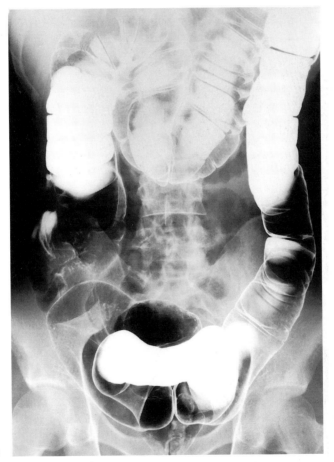

Fig. 5.10

This barium enema radiograph (Fig. 5.10) demonstrates a stricture involving the caecum. A magnified view (Fig. 5.11) identifies mucosal ulceration within the stricture (curved black arrow). The terminal ileum has been dragged superiorly due to extensive caecal scarring (white arrow).

This patient has ileocaecal tuberculosis (TB). The differential diagnosis includes Crohn's disease, malignancy (carcinoma and lymphoma) and other infective agents (actinomycosis and amoebiasis).

Features of gastrointestinal tract tuberculosis

• Rare in the Western world though increasing numbers of cases are being recorded.
• Increased risk in patients with HIV (human immunodeficiency virus).

The diagnosis may be confirmed by endoscopic biopsy specimens demonstrating caseating granulomas (tuberculin skin test is invariably negative). The ileocaecal segment is most commonly involved, presumably due to abundance of lymphoid tissue.

Mycobacterium tuberculosis, *M. bovis* and *M. intracellulare* are the usual organisms.

Approximately one third of patients present with tuberculous peritonitis.

Further reading

Balthazar, E.J., Gordon, R. & Hulnick, D. (1990) Ileocaecal tuberculosis: CT and radiologic evaluation. *American Journal of Roentgenology* **154**, 499–503.

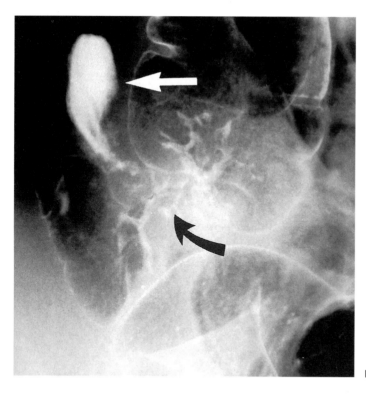

Fig. 5.11

CASE 7

This 54-year-old man presents with a fever and left-sided chest pain 6 weeks following a palliative left nephrectomy for extensive renal cell carcinoma.

What does this erect chest radiograph (Fig. 5.12) show?
What is the most likely cause of this finding?
What additional imaging will confirm your suspicion?

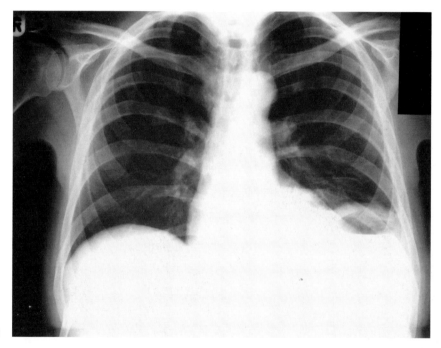

Fig. 5.12

This erect chest radiograph (Fig. 5.12) shows an abnormal air/fluid level beneath the left hemi-diaphragm. This fluid appears too lateral to be within the stomach, raising the suspicion of a subphrenic collection/abscess.

Radiographic features of an intra-abdominal abscess

• Small bubbles of gas outside bowel lumen, often unchanged on sequential films.
• Abnormal air/fluid level.
• Radiolucent bands (air) tracking along fascial planes.
• Loss of definition or displacement of abdominal viscera.
• Elevation of the diaphragm and/or pleural effusion.

Whilst a high proportion of intra-abdominal abscesses can be identified on radiographs, the diagnosis is usually made with ultrasound and/or CT. Contrast-enhanced CT imaging in this patient demonstrates a large collection of fluid and air in the left subphrenic space (Fig. 5.13, white arrow). Extensive residual renal cell carcinoma is highlighted (black arrow) in the left para-aortic region.

Ultrasound and CT imaging techniques have limited the role of radionuclide (technetium-labelled leucocyte or gallium) scanning in the diagnosis of intra-abdominal abscesses. This is in part due to a delay in the acquisition of images and insufficient resolution to guide needle drainage. This patient underwent percutaneous abscess drainage under CT imaging guidance.

Further reading

Halasz, N.A. (1970) Subphrenic abscess. Myths and facts. *Journal of the American Medical Association* **214**, 724–726.

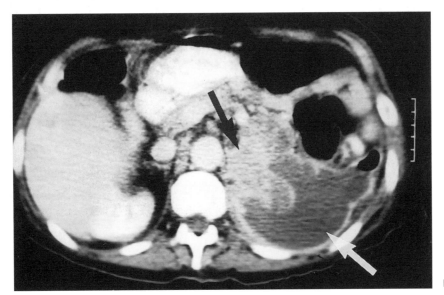

Fig. 5.13

CASE 8

This 80-year-old man presented with a history of intermittent right upper quadrant pain thought to be due to biliary colic. Ultrasound had shown a normal gall bladder. However, multiple complex cystic lesions were identified within the liver.

What is this investigation (Fig. 5.14)?
What does it show?
Could it be relevant to the patient's symptoms?

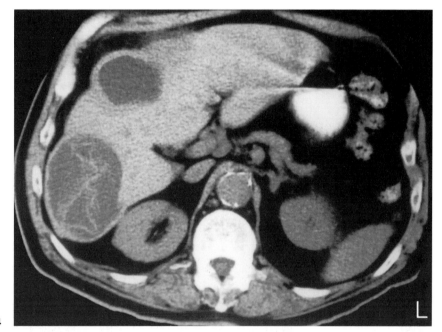

Fig. 5.14

Figure 5.14 is a CT image following oral contrast only through this patient's upper abdomen. Two cystic lesions are observed within the right lobe of the liver. The more posterior lesion distorts the liver capsule and is seen to contain serpiginous strands of soft tissue density. These features are characteristic of hydatid disease of the liver.

Hydatid disease is an endemic world-wide zoonosis caused by the larval stage of the echinococcus tapeworm. The most common human form is *Echinococcus granulosus*. Humans can develop the disease as an accidental intermediate host, e.g. by eating food contaminated by canine faeces containing larval eggs. The egg hatches in the duodenum allowing larvae to penetrate the intestinal wall and reach the portal circulation. It follows that the liver is the most common site of the disease, though no organ is exempt.

Imaging findings in hepatic hydatid disease

• Often multiple cysts, more common in the right lobe than the left.
• Complex cystic mass with multiple septations (a 'water-lily' sign as in this patient, Fig. 5.14).
• Pericystic calcification.

Complications of hepatic hydatid disease

• Infection.
• Intermittent biliary obstruction (as in this case) due to cyst communication with biliary tree.
• Cyst rupture.

Further reading

Lewall, D.B. (1998) Hydatid disease: biology, pathology, imaging and classification. *Clinical Radiology* **52**, 863–874.

CASE 9

This 65-year-old postmenopausal woman presents with a lump in the upper outer quadrant of the right breast.

What does the right oblique mammogram show (Fig. 5.15)?
What does the ultrasound of the right breast show (Fig. 5.16)?
What is the differential diagnosis?

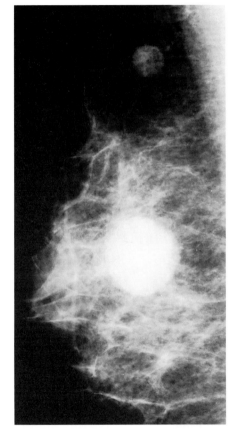

Fig. 5.15

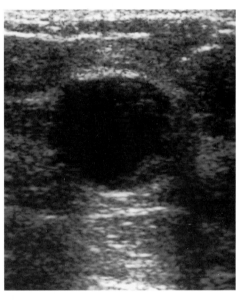

Fig. 5.16

The right oblique mammogram (Fig. 5.15) shows a 2.0-cm diameter mass with well-defined margins above the nipple. It was also visible on the craniocaudal view which confirmed its position to be in the upper outer quadrant, corresponding with the palpable abnormality. There is a normal intramammary node seen in the axillary region. The reproduced ultrasound image (Fig. 5.17) confirms a predominantly cystic lesion with well-defined margins and distal acoustic enhancement (white arrows). It does, however, have echogenic material peripherally (curved white arrow) and is therefore classified as a complex cyst. The lesion was surgically removed and found to be an intracystic papillary carcinoma.

Differential diagnosis of a complex cyst in the breast

The differential diagnosis of a complex cyst in the breast includes both benign and malignant lesions.
• Benign papilloma.
• Intracystic papillary carcinoma.
• Intracystic ductal carcinoma *in situ* (DCIS).
• Haemorrhage into a cyst. This may be spontaneous or following fine-needle aspiration (FNA).

FNA and core biopsy are unreliable in the evaluation of complex cystic lesions as it is impossible to exclude an intracystic papillary carcinoma without sampling the entire lesion. This diagnosis was indeed confirmed after complete surgical removal.

Ultrasound in investigation of breast disease

Indications for ultrasound in investigation of breast disease include:
• women under the age of 35 years with a lump or palpable change;
• as an adjunct to mammography in women over the age of 35 presenting with breast lumps;
• further characterization of mammographic abnormalities;
• mammographically dense breasts;
• assessment of pregnancy-related breast disease;
• evaluation of breast prostheses;
• guidance of FNA and core biopsy.

Ultrasound features of a simple cyst

• Absence of internal echoes.
• Well-defined margins.
• Acoustic enhancement distally. The sound beam is attenuated less by fluid than by solid tissue, causing an increase in the amplitude (brightness) of echoes distal to the cyst.

Further reading

Schneider, J.A. (1989) Invasive papillary breast carcinoma: mammographic and sonographic appearance. *Radiology* **171**, 377–379.

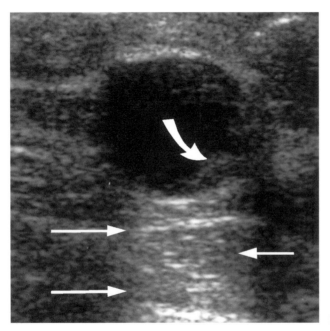

Fig. 5.17

CASE 10

This 72-year-old man presented with a lump behind the left nipple.

What does the left oblique mammogram show (Fig. 5.18)?
What does the left breast ultrasound show (Fig. 5.19)?
What is the diagnosis?

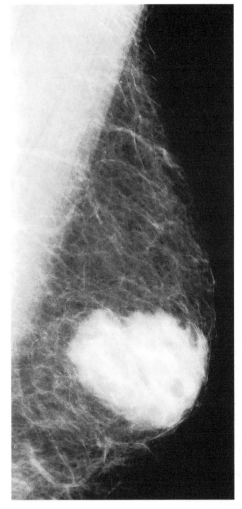

Fig. 5.18

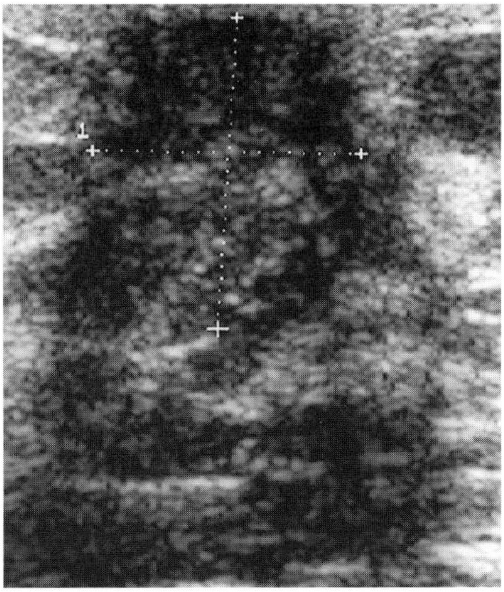

Fig. 5.19

The mammogram (Fig. 5.18) shows a 4 cm diameter poorly defined area of increased density centred behind the left nipple. There is no distortion of the surrounding breast stroma. Ultrasound confirms a 4 cm × 3 cm area of heterogeneous echogenicity with poorly defined margins in the left retro-areolar location (between callipers, Fig. 5.19). There is reduced transmission of sound through the lesion (the opposite of distal acoustic enhancement seen in cysts) and it is therefore solid.

The imaging appearances are characteristic of gynaecomastia.

Gynaecomastia is defined as an abnormal increase in the stromal and ductal components of the male breast. It is most common in men under 30 years of age and is usually idiopathic. It is thought to be caused by a hormonal imbalance with relevant excess of oestrogens. As a consequence the majority of cases occur at the times in life when there is a rapid physiological hormonal change (i.e. neonatally, at puberty and in the elderly who paradoxically exhibit decreasing testicular function).

Causes of gynaecomastia

- Idiopathic (rapid physiological hormonal change).
- Drugs (oestrogens, thiazides and digoxin).
- Liver disease (cirrhosis and hepatocellular carcinoma).
- Adrenal and testicular neoplasms.
- Chronic renal and pulmonary disease.

Gynaecomastia may be bilateral, and imaging in a young age group (less than 30 years) is usually inappropriate as a diagnosis is usually made on clinical grounds. However, a unilateral breast lump in older men should be investigated to exclude malignancy. Breast cancer is most common in men over the age of 60 years. In contrast to the ultrasound appearance (Fig. 5.19) of gynaecomastia, the image below (Fig. 5.20) shows features typical of a breast cancer in a man. A well-defined, lobulated and hypoechoic mass lies eccentric to the nipple.

Further reading

Stewart, R.A.L., Howlett, D.C. & Hearn, F.J. (1997) Pictorial review: the imaging features of male breast disease. *Clinical Radiology* **52**, 739–744.

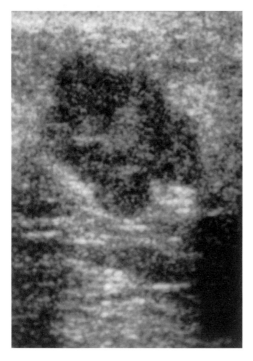

Fig. 5.20

CASE 11

This 48-year-old woman presents with a 3-month history of a rapidly growing lump in the upper portion of her right breast.

What does the right craniocaudal mammogram show (Fig. 5.21)?
What does the right breast ultrasound show (Fig. 5.22)?
What is the most likely diagnosis?

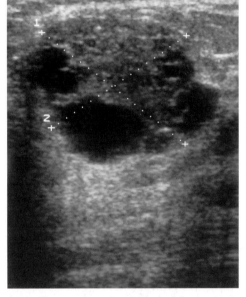

Fig. 5.22

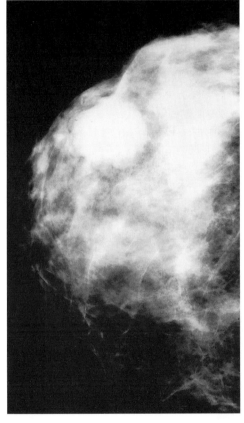

Fig. 5.21

The right craniocaudal mammogram (Fig. 5.21) shows an approximately 3-cm diameter lobulated mass with well-defined margins. The oblique mammogram (not shown) confirmed its position in the upper central breast.

The ultrasound (Fig. 5.22, reproduced on this page as Fig. 5.23) shows a 2.8 cm × 2.6 cm diameters predominantly solid mass (between callipers). It has a lobulated contour with well-defined margins. There are several cystic areas within the mass (white arrows) as well as hyperechoic septations (curved white arrow). The mass does demonstrate a slight increase in through transmission of sound, presumably related to its partially cystic nature (see Case 9 in this chapter).

The clinical presentation and radiological features are strongly suggestive of a phyllodes tumour. As malignant change must be excluded, the patient underwent a local excision. Histological analysis confirmed a benign phyllodes tumour.

Phyllodes tumour (giant fibroadenoma, adenosarcoma or cystosarcoma phyllodes)

- Rare, comprising 1.5% of all breast tumours.
- Women are usually in their fifth or sixth decades.
- Presents as a rapidly enlarging breast lump.
- Benign form of intracanalicular fibroadenoma.
- Tendency to recur locally if excision is incomplete. Malignant conversion occurs in 5–10%.

Ultrasound features suggestive of malignancy in a solid breast lump

- Heterogeneous echogenicity.
- Hypoechoic relative to adjacent normal tissue.
- Irregular margins and an echogenic rim of variable thickness.
- Posterior acoustic shadowing.
- Long-axis orientation perpendicular to skin.

Further reading

Moffat, C.J.C., Tinder, S.E., Dixon, A.R., Elston, C.W., Blamey, R.W. & Ellis, I.O. (1995) Phyllodes tumours of the breast: a clinico-pathological review of 32 cases. *Histopathology* **27**, 205–218.

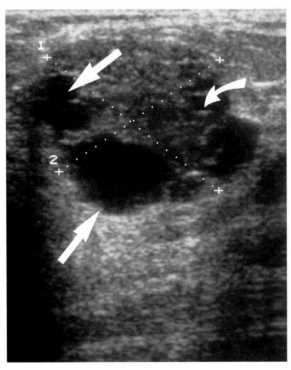

Fig. 5.23

CASE 12

This 36-year-old woman presents with a 2-month history of a left breast lump.

What do the left craniocaudal mammogram (Fig. 5.24) and left breast ultrasound (Fig. 5.25) show?
What is the diagnosis?

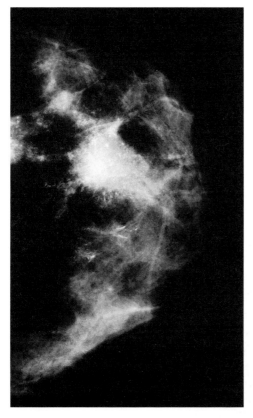

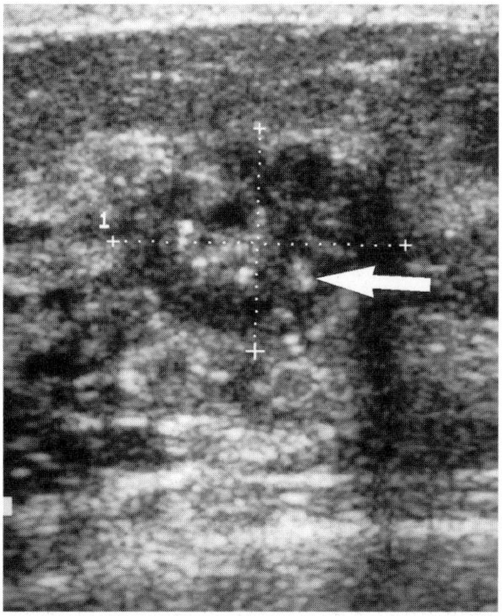

Fig. 5.25

Fig. 5.24

In Fig. 5.24 there is a 2-cm spiculated opacity lying centrally in the breast. There are also extensive microcalcifications which on closer inspection have marked variability in form, size and density, resembling 'fine grains of salt'. Ultrasound examination of the palpable lesion (Fig. 5.25) demonstrates an irregular, hypoechoic mass corresponding with the mammographic lesion (between callipers) which contains internal microcalcifications (white arrow).

Fine-needle aspiration of the solid lump revealed malignant cells and subsequent surgical resection (mastectomy and axillary sampling) confirmed an invasive ductal carcinoma arising within an extensive area of ductal carcinoma *in situ* (DCIS).

Ductal carcinoma *in situ*

- Increasing incidence with advancing age.
- Two types.

High-grade DCIS ('comedo type')
Sixty per cent of all DCIS. Usually show the typical malignant-type microcalcifications on mammograms.

Low-grade DCIS ('non-comedo type')
Forty per cent of all DCIS. May show typical malignant-type microcalcifications. However, the size of 'non-comedo' DCIS is often underestimated mammographically. May be mammographically occult.

Between 20 and 50% of patients with DCIS will develop invasive breast cancer within 10 years of initial diagnosis.

A magnified image (Fig. 5.26) of a left craniocaudal mammogram in another patient demonstrates typical malignant ductal calcifications in more detail.

Malignant microcalcifications

Form
- *Granular*: small, dot-like and clustered together to resemble 'fine grains of salt'.
- *Casting*: microcalcifications take the form of 'casts' of segments of the ductal lumen, often exhibiting a branching pattern.

Size
Wide range though the distribution is intraductal.

Density
Wide variability.

Distribution
Usually clustered within an area of the breast, often within one lobe.

Further reading

Tabar, L. & Dean, P. (1985) *Teaching Atlas of Mammography*, 2nd edn. Thième Verlag, Stuttgart.

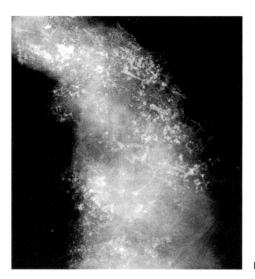

Fig. 5.26

CHAPTER 6

Sheila C. Rankin

CASE 1

A 40-year-old female presents with recurrent episodes of acute left flank pain with associated microscopic haematuria.

What does the unenhanced CT image (Fig. 6.1) show?
What is the likely diagnosis?

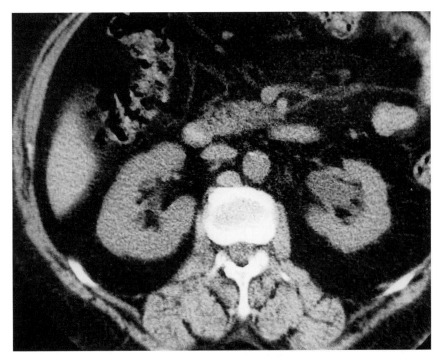

Fig. 6.1

The axial CT image (Fig. 6.1) demonstrates dilatation of the renal pelvis on the left.

This is due to obstruction to the left kidney which, in view of the history, is likely to be due to recurrent ureteric calculi. Ureteric tumour is possible but less likely.

Acute flank pain is extremely common. The intravenous urogram (IVU) is used for the diagnosis of renal calculi and can identify the size and site of the calculus and assess function and the degree of obstruction to the kidney. Unenhanced spiral CT does provide an alternative modality for the investigation of renal colic.

CT imaging for detection of ureteric calculi

Advantages
• High sensitivity, specificity and accuracy for diagnosis (97%, 96% and 97%, respectively).
• More rapid than IVU, no delayed films and the avoidance of potentially nephrotoxic contrast.
• Able to demonstrate extraurinary causes for acute flank pain: appendicitis, ovarian pathology, diverticulitis, colonic neoplasm and cholecystitis.

• Images can be reformatted to obtain better demonstration.

Disadvantages
• Increased radiation dose compared with IVU.
• No functional data.
• Degree of obstruction may be difficult to assess.

A reformatted coronal (CT) image (Fig. 6.2) shows calculus in the lower left ureter (arrowhead) with dilated pelvis and proximal ureter (open arrow).

Apart from identifying the calculus in the ureter, CT also demonstrates the secondary signs of ureteric calculi, including hydronephrosis, hydroureter, increased renal size and perinephric stranding. Interestingly, the extent of stranding is proportional to the degree of obstruction.

Further reading

Smith, R.C., Levine, J. & Rosenfeld, A.T. (1999) Helical CT of urinary tract stones. *Radiologic Clinics of North America* **37**, 911–952.

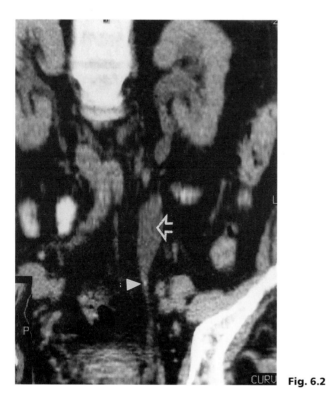

Fig. 6.2

CASE 2

A 30-year-old man involved in a road traffic accident presents with abdominal bruising and left loin tenderness on palpation. Haematuria was noted.

CT imaging of the abdomen was performed using intravenous contrast medium.

What does the contrast-enhanced CT image (Fig. 6.3) show?
What is the diagnosis?

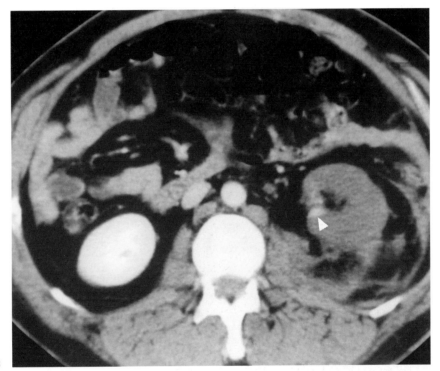

Fig. 6.3

The CT image (Fig. 6.3), demonstrates that the right kidney appears normal and is excreting contrast. There is no evidence of enhancement of the left kidney, apart from a small amount peripherally and medially (arrowhead).

The lack of enhancement of the left kidney would be compatible with renal artery occlusion. A further more cranial axial section (Fig. 6.4) confirms thrombus within the left renal artery (white arrowhead) and renal vein (black arrow). Note the perinephric haematoma (open arrow).

Renal artery trauma

• Follows deceleration injury or blunt trauma.
• Stretching/shearing forces on the renal artery cause intimal tears progressing to thrombosis and occlusion.

• Infarction may be segmental or complete.
• Absent/partial nephrogram on CT. Occasional peripheral rim enhancement due to capsular arterial supply.

Patients with renal trauma who are not shocked and have normal renal function can be managed conservatively. Severe disruption of the renal pedicle with profuse bleeding and compromised renal function requires emergency laparotomy. In this group reconstruction is often impractical and a nephrectomy is necessary. Radiologically guided embolization may be considered if arterial extravasation is seen on contrast-enhanced CT imaging.

Further reading

Novelline, R.A., Rhea, J.T. & Bell, T. (1999) Helical CT of abdominal trauma. *Radiologic Clinics of North America* **37**, 591–612.

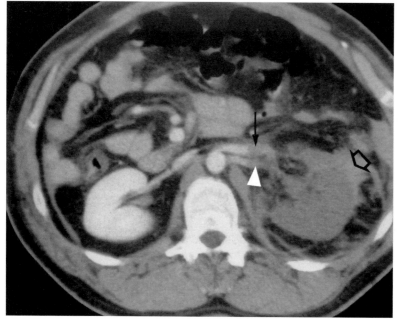

Fig. 6.4

CASE 3

A 10-year-old boy presents with mild upper abdominal tenderness having fallen off a swing. On ultrasound a small amount of intraperitoneal fluid was seen. The spleen was not well visualized. CT imaging of his abdomen was performed.

What abnormality is highlighted (arrowhead) on the contrast-enhanced CT image (Fig. 6.5)?

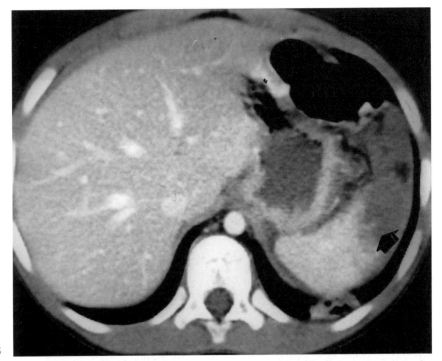

Fig. 6.5

The axial contrast-enhanced CT image (Fig. 6.5) reveals extensive laceration of the spleen with associated haematoma (arrowhead).

The spleen is the most frequently injured organ in patients who have suffered blunt abdominal trauma. Lower rib fractures suggest this injury, although an intact rib cage does not rule out splenic trauma. CT imaging can accurately diagnose splenic trauma though the actual extent is frequently underestimated. Moreover, CT imaging cannot predict which patients can be treated conservatively.

Trauma is a leading cause of death in men and women aged less than 40 years of age. Approximately 10% of all trauma deaths are due to abdominal injuries.

Mechanism of injury

Blunt
Compression, shearing or deceleration forces.

Penetrating
• Stab wounds cause tissue damage by laceration.
• High-velocity rifle wounds transfer more kinetic energy, causing damage by cavitation and fragmentation.

Further reading

McKenney, K.L. (1999) Ultrasound of blunt abdominal trauma. *Radiologic Clinics of North America* **37**, 879–893.

Diagnostic studies in blunt trauma

	Diagnostic peritoneal lavage	Ultrasound	CT imaging
Diagnosis	Early	Early	Delayed
Sensitivity	98%	85–90%	90–95%
Specificity	Poor	Intermediate	Good
Eligibility	All patients	All patients	Haemodynamically stable patients
Pitfalls	Invasive and negative for retroperitoneal structures	Operator dependent Negative in obese patients and in the presence of excessive bowel gas	Irradiation and patient co-operation

CASE 4

A 60-year-old man presents in hypovolaemic shock with abdominal distension. He is found to be anaemic.

What abnormalities are present on the supine abdominal radiograph (Fig. 6.6)?
Suggest a differential diagnosis.
What investigations would confirm your diagnosis?

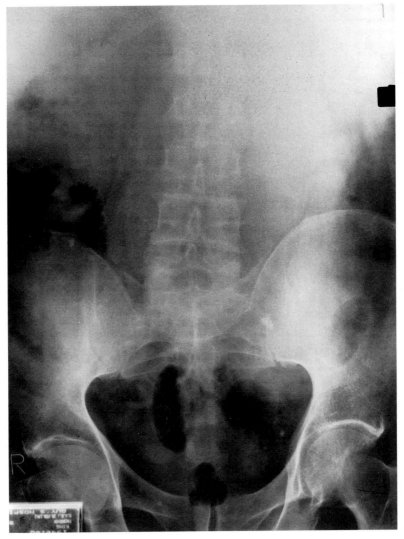

Fig. 6.6

On the abdominal radiograph (Fig. 6.6) there is no evidence of large or small bowel distension. The right psoas shadow is well seen but the left is not, and there is an impression of a mass in the left flank, displacing bowel laterally. The underlying spine appears normal.

Loss of psoas shadow on plain abdominal radiograph

Inability to see one of the psoas shadows may be normal. If previously visualized then consider retroperitoneal pathology including:
• Psoas abscess, which may be associated with spinal or intra-abdominal infection.
• Bleeding abdominal aortic aneurysm. With this patient's history suggesting sudden blood loss, this is the most likely diagnosis.
• Large renal tumour involving the psoas with obliteration of fat planes.

Further investigations can include ultrasound to assess the aorta and retroperitoneum although the presence of bowel gas may render the images suboptimal. MR imaging can visualize the aorta and retroperitoneum but may not be readily available. In the stable patient, contrast-enhanced CT imaging is the investigation of choice. The postcontrast CT image (Fig. 6.7)

shows an aneurysm of the abdominal aorta (arrow). There is perfusion of the right kidney. A large soft tissue mass in the retroperitoneum is compatible with a retroperitoneal bleed from the aneurysm (open arrow). Dramatically, contrast is seen leaking from the aneurysm into the retroperitoneal structures (arrowheads), indicating an acute ongoing bleed requiring emergency intervention.

Key CT features in the investigation of an abdominal aortic aneurysm

• Accurate assessment of size and extent.
• Relationship to renal arteries and iliac vessels.
• Length of aneurysmal neck.
• Aneurysmal wall thickness and the presence of any localized saccular dilatation.
• Assessment of coexistent, occlusive or aneurysmal arterial disease elsewhere.
• Exclusion of other abdominal pathology.

Further reading

Simoni, G., Perrone, R., Cittadini, G. *et al.* (1996) Helical CT for the study of abdominal aortic aneurysm in patients undergoing conventional surgical repair. *European Journal of Vascular and Endovascular Surgery* **12**, 354–358.

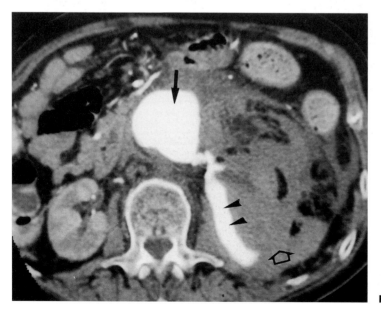

Fig. 6.7

CASE 5

A 44-year-old woman presents with progressive abdominal distension and discomfort.

What does the supine abdominal radiograph (Fig. 6.8) show?
What do the arrowheads indicate?
What further investigation could be performed?

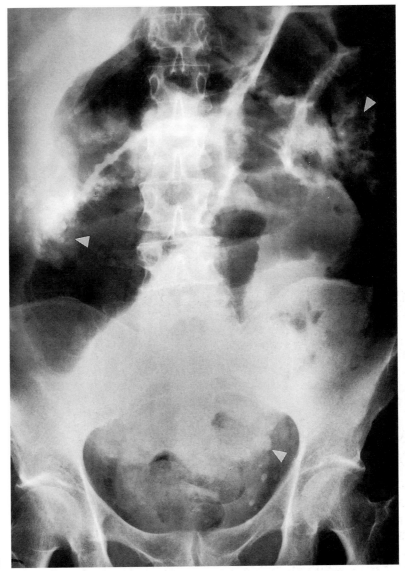

Fig. 6.8

The supine abdominal radiograph (Fig. 6.8) shows dilated loops of small bowel in the centre of the abdomen. There is calcification within the pelvis on the left and in the periphery of the abdomen on the right, as well as in the left upper quadrant (arrowheads), not conforming to the renal tract or gall bladder. CT imaging post oral contrast only (Fig. 6.9) indicates that the calcification is peritoneal. Peritoneal deposits in relation to the ascending colon are demonstrated (arrows). These were due to metastatic ovarian carcinoma.

CT imaging in ovarian cancer

• Multiloculated, cystic and solid tumours, commonly bilateral.
• Cysts with thick walls and internal septations.
• Heterotrophic calcification.
• Enables accurate staging, particularly of liver metastases and retroperitoneal lymphadeno-pathy. Large and small bowel, peritoneum and ureters may be secondarily involved. Small peritoneal deposits, particularly in the absence of ascites, may be missed.
• Overall sensitivity for detecting recurrent disease approaches 85%. Follow-up CA-125 levels should be used.
• Ovarian metastases from stomach or colon (Krukenberg tumours) have a very similar appearance.

Further reading

Kurtz, A.B., Tsimikas, J.V., Tempany, C.M. *et al.* (1999) Diagnosis and staging of ovarian cancer: comparative values of Doppler and conventional US, CT, and MR imaging correlated with surgery and histopathologic analysis—report of the Radiology Diagnostic Oncology Group. *Radiology* **212**, 19–27.

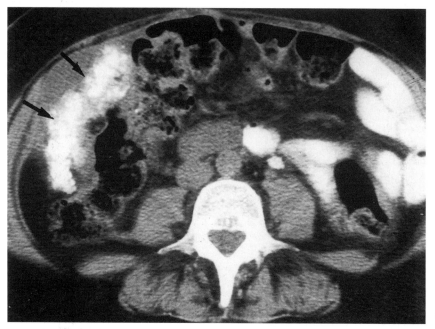

Fig. 6.9

CASE 6

An 80-year-old female presents with colicky abdominal pain and vomiting. A supine abdominal radiograph (Fig. 6.10) was obtained.

What are the radiological findings?
What is the diagnosis?

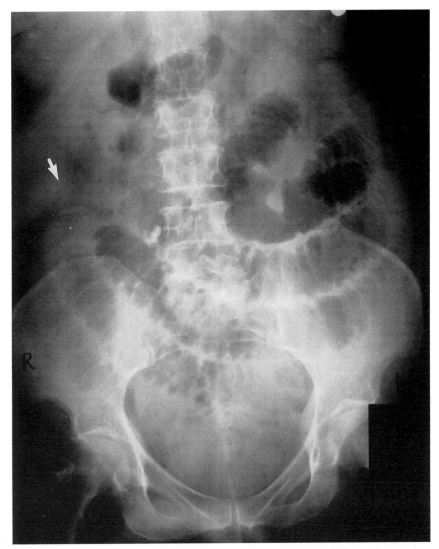

Fig. 6.10

On the abdominal radiograph there are three key findings:
- multiple, gas-filled loops of dilated small bowel consistent with small bowel obstruction;
- irregularly branching gas shadows present in the right upper quadrant which do not extend to the liver edge and represent air within the biliary tree;
- a rounded, calcific density which can just be visualized in the right mid-abdomen (arrowed) and represents an obstructing gallstone within the small bowel.

This patient has gallstone ileus.

Gallstone ileus

- Occurs in chronic cholecystitis with erosion of a gallstone into the gastrointestinal tract.
- Represents up to 25% of obstructions in patients over 70 years.
- Stones need to be quite large (> 2 cm) to cause obstruction, with the terminal ileum the most common site of stone impaction.
- There is a classic triad of imaging features described above. The presence of biliary tree air is variable and gallstone visualization depends on the degree of calcification.
- Change in position of a previously noted gallstone may provide a useful clue, as in this case. A previous right upper quadrant radiograph demonstrates the calcified gallstone (Fig. 6.11, arrow) and this has clearly migrated by the time of patient presentation (Fig. 6.10).
- Surgical enterotomy, with removal of the gallstone and relief of obstruction, will usually suffice.

Other causes of biliary tree air

- Patulous sphincter in elderly people.
- Post surgery or sphincterotomy.
- Biliary fistula secondary to malignancy or duodenal ulcer.

Further reading

Zoman, R.K. (2000) Cholelithiasis and cholecystitis In: *Textbook of Gastrointestinal Radiology* (eds R.M. Gore & M.S. Levine), 2nd edn, pp. 1335–1336. W.B. Saunders Co., Philadelphia.

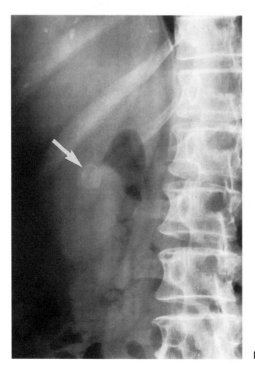

Fig. 6.11

CASE 7

A 7-year-old boy presents with acute abdominal pain and vomiting.

What does the supine abdominal radiograph (Fig. 6.12) show?
What does the arrow demonstrate?
What is the diagnosis?
What other radiological investigations can be used for this condition?

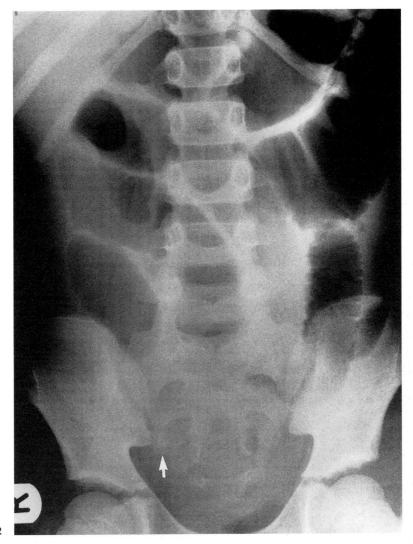

Fig. 6.12

The supine abdominal radiograph (Fig. 6.12) shows dilated loops of air-filled bowel. Valvulae conniventes are noted running across the bowel in the left flank, indicating that this is small bowel dilatation. The transverse colon is also dilated. There is a laminated calculus in the right iliac fossa close to the lower end of the right sacroiliac joint (arrow).

The radiological features are those of an ileus with an appendicolith in the right pelvis. The diagnosis is that of acute appendicitis.

Ultrasound and CT imaging have recently been used in the evaluation of patients with suspected appendicitis. Graded compression ultrasound is an excellent examination for children and thin adults, but is more difficult to perform in large patients.

Ultrasound criteria for the diagnosis of appendicitis

• Non-compressible distended appendix.
• Surrounding hypoechoic thickened wall greater than 2 mm in diameter.

• Maximum appendiceal diameter greater than 6 mm.
• Loculated pericolic fluid may be seen.
• Appendicolith seen in 30% of acute appendicitis.
• Reported sensitivity 77%, specificity 94% and accuracy 89%.

The entire appendix must be visualized before it can be called normal. Ultrasound will miss a retrocaecal appendicitis due to overlying gas.

CT imaging has the advantage that it is not operator dependent and will identify other causes of right-sided abdominal pain. In practice it is not widely used in the diagnosis of acute appendicitis. However, the CT image (Fig. 6.13) demonstrates typical changes highlighting appendiceal wall thickening (black arrow) with the diameter of the appendix greater than 6 mm.

Further reading

Rao, P.M., Rhea, J.T. & Novelline, R.A. (1999) Helical CT of appendicitis and diverticulitis. *Radiologic Clinics of North America* **37**, 895–910.

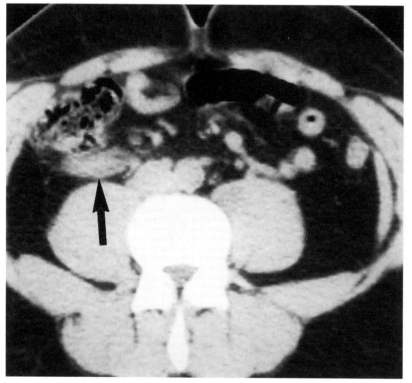

Fig. 6.13

CASE 8

A 70-year-old man presents with a history of intermittent bloody diar-rhoea complicated by the sudden onset of abdominal pain.

What does the supine abdominal radiograph (Fig. 6.14) show?
What feature is highlighted (arrow)?
What is the most likely aetiology and how may it be confirmed radiologically?

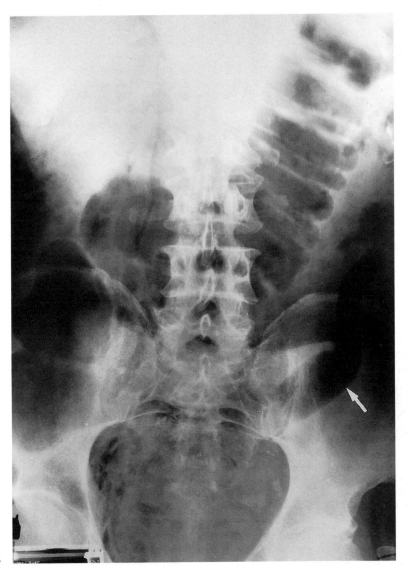

Fig. 6.14

The supine abdominal radiograph (Fig. 6.14) shows evidence of marked dilatation of the transverse colon with a narrowed and abnormal-appearing descending colon (arrow). There are streaks of air with linear gas collections along the right pelvic side wall extending up the psoas (pneumoretroperitoneum).

Retroperitoneal gas

- Bounded by fascial planes.
- Collects in a linear fashion along the psoas margins and renal outlines and under the medial surfaces of the hemidiaphragm.
- Sources include retroperitoneal portions of bowel (duodenum, ascending and descending colon, rectum).

Air from duodenal perforations tends to stay in the right pararenal space, whereas gas from the rectum may be limited to the perirectal space or involve all of the retroperitoneum extending up into the mediastinum! Gas from the sigmoid colon extends laterally along the margin of the psoas muscle and is the most likely source of pneumoretroperitoneum in this case.

Differential diagnosis of sigmoid perforation

- Diverticulitis.
- Ulcerative colitis/Crohn's disease.
- Rectosigmoid neoplasm.
- Trauma/instrumentation.

CT imaging may help differentiate inflammatory bowel disease from diverticulitis and carcinoma. In the CT image (Fig. 6.15) from this patient an abnormally thickened, narrowed, tubular sigmoid colon (white arrow) with no evidence of diverticula is noted. Air in the retroperitoneum (black arrows) and dilatation of the ascending colon (white open arrow) is evident. The diagnosis is of a perforation secondary to ulcerative colitis.

Further reading

Balthazor, E.J. (1991) CT of the gastrointestinal tract: principles and interpretation. *American Journal of Roentgenolgy* **156**, 23–32.

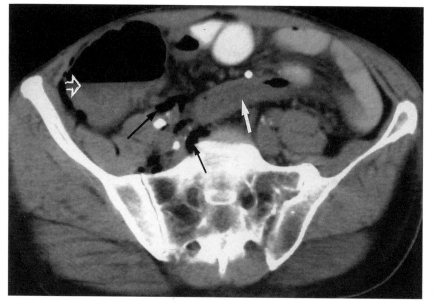

Fig. 6.15

CHAPTER 6

CASE 9

A 76-year-old man presents with chronic diarrhoea and episodes of flushing.

What does the contrast-enhanced CT image (Fig. 6.16) show?
What is a likely diagnosis?
What tests could you do to confirm the diagnosis?

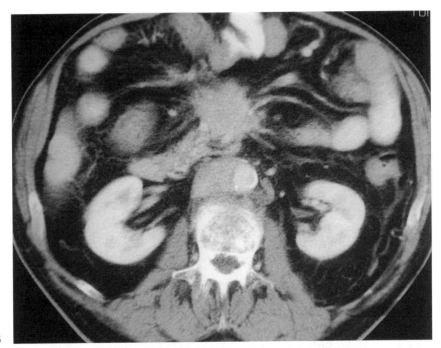

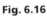 **Fig. 6.16**

The reproduced contrast-enhanced CT image (Fig. 6.17) highlights a mass in the mesentery (black arrow) with curvilinear strands extending towards surrounding bowel loops (white arrow). These represent thickened neurovascular bundles. There is thickening of the wall of the adjacent bowel loops (curved white arrow). There are enlarged para-aortic lymph nodes (curved black arrow).

The most likely diagnosis is carcinoid. In view of the diarrhoea and flushing this patient has carcinoid syndrome which is invariably associated with liver metastasis. The thickening of the bowel loops, seen on these CT images, relates to a desmoplastic reaction caused by the local action of serotonin. Once this occurs 50–85% will have nodal metastases. Liver metastases in carcinoid are hypervascular and best identified during the hepatic arterial phase soon after the injection of intravenous contrast medium.

Carcinoid tumours

- Fifty per cent occur in the appendix.
- More common in the ileum than jejunum, accounting for 30% of all small bowel neoplasms.
- Eighty per cent of tumours greater than 2 cm will have metastatic disease.
- Often multiple and may be associated with metachronous malignancies (30% of patients).
- Carcinoid syndrome associated with hepatic metastases in 95% of patients.

Urine 5-HIAA (5-hydroxyindoleacetic acid) levels and plasma serotonin levels will be elevated. Indium octreotide nuclear medicine imaging is very helpful for both diagnosis and therapy.

Further reading

Memon, M.A. & Nelson, H. (1997) Gastrointestinal carcinoid tumours: current management strategies. *Diseases of the Colon and Rectum* **40**, 1101–1118.

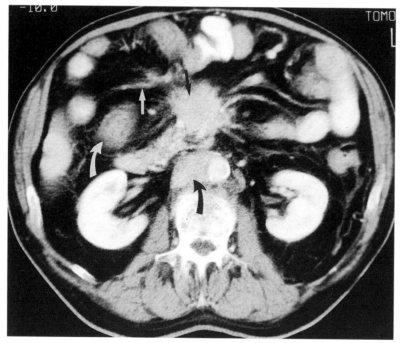

Fig. 6.17

CASE 10

A 60-year-old man with a previous history of pancreatitis presents with a palpable, pulsatile epigastric mass. CT imaging of the upper abdomen was performed following oral and intravenous contrast medium.

What does this CT image (Fig. 6.18) show?
What abnormality is highlighted (arrowheads)?
What is the diagnosis?
What other complications can occur in this condition?

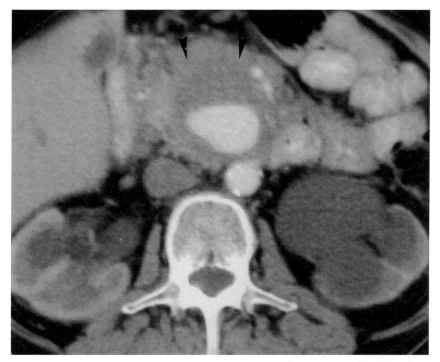

Fig. 6.18

The CT image (Fig. 6.18) shows a well-defined enhancing mass of equal intensity to the aorta lying posteriorly. It is surrounded by a soft tissue mass (arrowheads). Note is also made of a coincidental left hydronephrosis.

The appearances are of a pseudoaneurysm of the superior mesenteric artery developing secondary to acute pancreatitis. The treatment is radiological with embolization of the aneurysm.

Causes of acute pancreatitis

• *Obstruction.* Gallstones, stenosis, duodenum diverticulum, afferent loop obstruction.
• *Toxic and metabolic.* Alcohol, drugs, hypertriglyceridaemia, hypocalcaemia, scorpion sting.
• *Trauma.*
• *Iatrogenic.* Post endoscopic retrograde cholangiopancreatography.
• *Infections.* Mumps virus, Coxsackie virus, *Mycoplasma.*
• *Others.* Ischaemia, tumour, autoimmune disease.

The clinical diagnosis of pancreatitis may be difficult. Although the serum amylase level is the single most useful laboratory test it may not always be elevated. The pancreas is the only known source of lipase and serum assays for this are a putative marker for pancreatitis.

Radiological imaging, although an insensitive index of acute pancreatitis, can be important in confirming the diagnosis and assist in the early detection of complications. On ultrasound the pancreas appears diffusely enlarged and hypoechoic. Local phlegmons or fluid collections may be identified; however, overlying gas often precludes accurate visualization with ultrasound. Currently CT imaging is the investigation of choice. Ideally the accrual of information is gained after oral contrast and both before and after intravenous contrast effusion, which specifically highlights pancreatic viability. Patchy areas of non-enhancement following intravenous contrast indicate pancreatic necrosis. Gas bubbles are strongly suggestive of abscess formation and phlegmons are masses of inflammatory tissue. Pseudocysts are clearly visualized.

Local complications of pancreatitis

• Pseudocysts.
• Inflammatory mass (phlegmon) and abscess formation.
• Pseudoaneurysm formation.
• Splenic and portal vein thrombosis.
• Obstructive jaundice.

Further reading

Dalzell, D.P., Scharling, E.S., Ott, D.J. & Wolfman, N.T. (1998) Acute pancreatitis: the role of diagnostic imaging [review]. *Critical Reviews in Diagnostic Imaging* **39**, 339–363.

CASE 11

A 54-year-old diabetic man presented, unwell with urinary tract infection.

What abnormality is highlighted (arrows) on the supine abdominal radiograph (Fig. 6.19)?

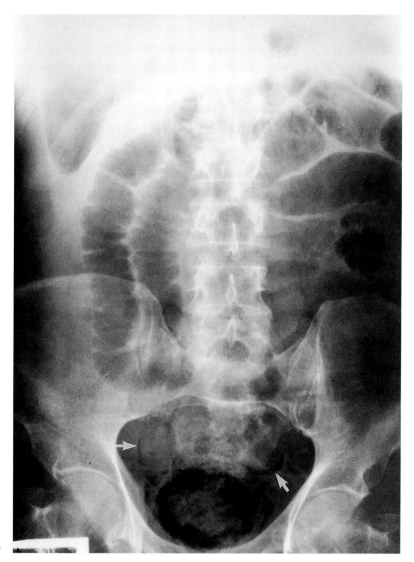

Fig. 6.19

The supine abdominal radiograph (Fig. 6.19) reveals an abnormal gas shadow overlying the pelvis corresponding to gas within the bladder. On closer inspection linear gas shadows extend superiorly along the path of both lower ureters (arrows) and moreover there are bubbles of gas within the bladder wall. Note is also made of dilated loops of small bowel.

This man is diabetic and the diagnosis is emphysematous pyelonephritis.

Emphysematous pyelonephritis

• Fulminant necrotizing infection of the kidney and perirenal tissues.
• Due to *Escherichia coli* (68%), *Klebsiella* (9%).
• Immunocompromised patients, especially diabetics, are vulnerable.
• Rarely bilateral.

• Overall mortality is greatly reduced where nephrectomy accompanies antibiotic therapy.

Contrast-enhanced CT imaging (Fig. 6.20) of the same patient shows gas in the renal pelvis on the right (black arrow) with gas in the renal parenchyma on both sides. There is patchy enhancement bilaterally with wedge-shaped areas of non-enhancement (black arrowheads) secondary to infarction. Subcapsular fluid is also evident (white arrow).

Further reading

Kawashima, A. Sandler, C.M., Ernst, R.D., Goldman, S.M., Raval, B. & Fishman, E.K. (1997) Renal inflammatory disease: the current role of CT [review]. *Critical Reviews in Diagnostic Imaging* **38**, 369–415.

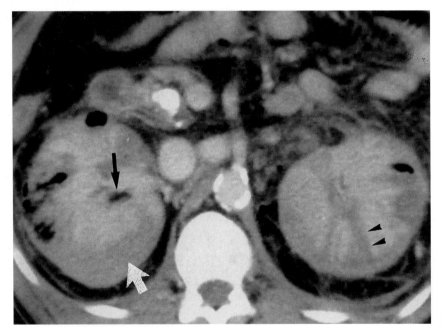

Fig. 6.20

CASE 12

A 55-year-old woman presents with upper abdominal pain, anorexia and weight loss.

What does the contrast-enhanced CT image (Fig. 6.21) of the pancreatic region demonstrate?
What is the diagnosis?

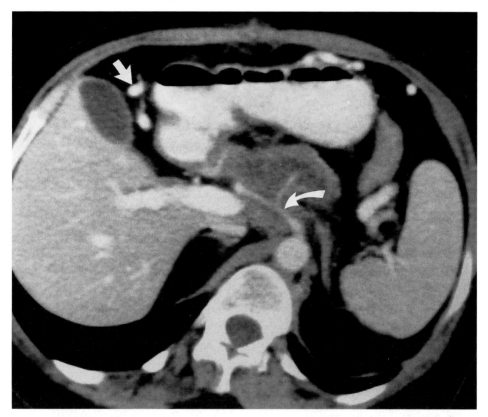

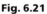
Fig. 6.21

A CT image (Fig. 6.21) reveals an irregular soft tissue mass in the region of the pancreatic head surrounding the coeliac axis (curved white arrow). Prominent collateral vessels around the stomach (white arrow) are indicative of splenic vein thrombosis. On a more caudal image (Fig. 6.22) the superior mesenteric vein (black arrowhead) is surrounded and invaded by the mass. Moreover, tumour infiltrates around the right crus of the diaphragm (open arrow). There is no evidence of intrahepatic biliary duct dilatation.

The radiological features are those of carcinoma of the pancreas with vascular invasion. By these criteria, it is inoperable.

Pancreatic adenocarcinoma

- Occurs in 10 per 100 000 population.
- Risk factors include tobacco, diabetes, alcohol and family history.
- Sixty-five per cent of tumours arise within the head of the pancreas.
- At diagnosis 85% of cases are either locally advanced or accompanied by metastases.
- Less than 5% 5-year survival rate.

Ultrasound and CT imaging are the two methods most frequently used to confirm a clinical suspicion of pancreatic cancer. Both can demonstrate pancreatic masses, dilatation of pancreatic and bile ducts, hepatic metastases and extrapancreatic spread. On ultrasound pancreatic tumours appear less echogenic than the surrounding parenchyma. On enhanced CT imaging they are typically of lower attenuation than normal pancreas. CT imaging has a higher sensitivity, approaching 70%, compared to that of ultrasound. MR imaging confers no additional advantage.

Accurate preoperative staging can select potentially resectable tumours and avoids inappropriate surgery. Both CT and MR imaging are poor at predicting resectability since microscopic spread will be missed and specificity for lymph node metastases is poor. Laparoscopy will show evidence of hepatic or peritoneal spread even when CT imaging is negative. Angiography offers additional valuable preoperative knowledge on the vascular anatomy of patients.

Further reading

Stanley, R.J & Semelka, R.C. (1998) Pancreas. In: *Computed Body Tomography with MRI Correlation*, (eds J.K.T. Lee, S.S. Sagel, R.J. Stanley & J.P. Heiken), 3rd edn, pp. 873–959. Lippincott-Raven, Philadelphia.

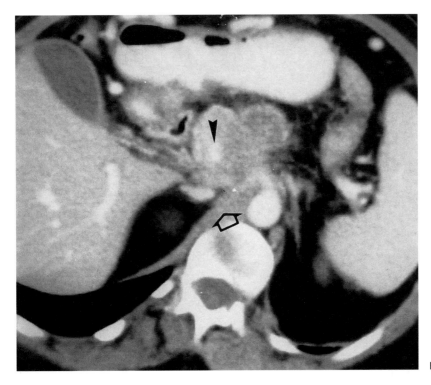

Fig. 6.22

CHAPTER 7

Elizabeth Ruffell

CASE 1

A 70-year-old female patient presents with several days' history of severe epigastric pain and vomiting.

What abnormal features are seen on the plain abdominal radiograph (Fig. 7.1)?

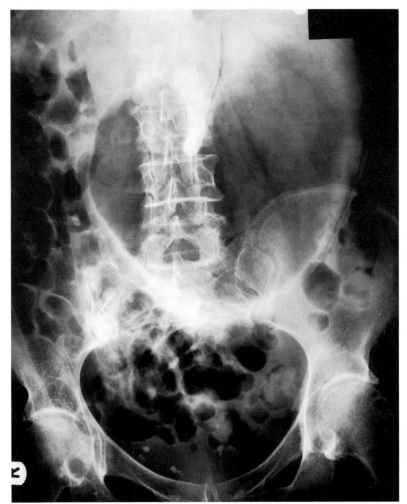

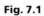

Fig. 7.1

The abdominal radiograph (Fig. 7.1) shows marked gastric distension with linear gas in the wall of the stomach. The gas is running deep to and parallel with the mucosal surface of the stomach. Ischaemic change or infarction of the gastric wall as a result of gastric outlet obstruction has caused these appearances.

Causes of gastric outlet obstruction in adults

• Peptic ulceration (as in this case).
• Carcinoma (primary gastric, pancreatic or secondary extrinsic compression by metastatic lymphadenopathy).
• Volvulus.
• Crohn's disease.
• Intersussception of tumour or mucosa.
• Ingestion of caustic substances causing stricture formation.

Intramural gas can take the form of a linear or cystic (blebs) pattern. Linear tracking of gas often accompany visceral distension where mucosal defects allow gas entry. The presence of gas in the bowel wall does not necessarily indicate irreversible ischaemia and its presence should be correlated with the clinical state of the patient.

Causes of intestinal intramural gas

1 Linear pattern associated with ischaemia or infarction.
   • Mesenteric vascular disease.
   • Obstruction.
   • Toxic colon, e.g. colitis or necrotizing enterocolitis.
2 Linear gas without infarction.
   • Connective tissue disorders, e.g. scleroderma.
   • Caustic ingestion.
   • Iatrogenic, e.g. post-surgery catheterization, stenting, endoscopic biopsy.
   • Immunosuppression.
3 Cystic gas pattern.
   • Pneumatosis cystoides intestinalis.
   • Associated with chronic obstructive lung disease.

Further reading

Pear, B.L. (1998) Pneumatosis intestinalis: a review. *Radiology* **207**, 13–19.

CASE 2

An erect chest film (Fig. 7.2) taken immediately postoperatively.

Describe the changes seen on the film.
What action should be taken to rectify the problem?

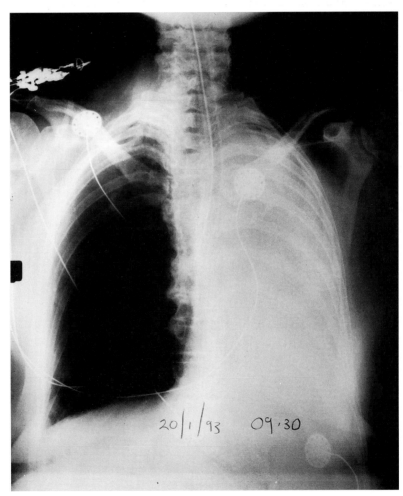

20/1/93   09·30

Fig. 7.2

The chest radiograph (Fig. 7.2) reveals opacity of the left hemithorax with shift of the mediastinum to the left. There is loss of clarity of the left mediastinal border and of the left hemidiaphragm. The tip of the endo-tracheal tube lies in the right main bronchus. There is collapse of the left lung secondary to malpositioning of the endo-tracheal tube.

The endo-tracheal tube should be withdrawn so that its tip lies above the carina.

Its corrected position and full re-expansion of the left lung can be confirmed by a repeat erect chest radiograph (Fig. 7.3). In this second radiograph the mediastinal and diaphragmatic borders on the left are now clearly visible as aerated lung forms a natural contrast. This is referred to as a 'silhouette' sign.

A loss of clarity of part of the mediastinal or diaphragmatic border indicates pathology either in the adjacent pleura or in the adjacent lung segment.

Further reading

Felson, B., MD. (1973) Localization of intrathoracic lesions. In: *Chest Roentgenology*, pp. 22–60. W.B. Saunders Co., Philadelphia.

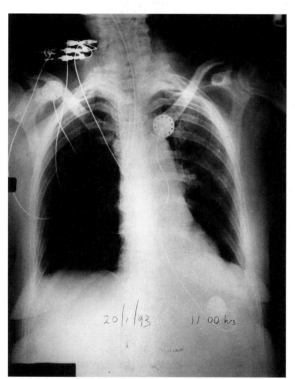

Fig. 7.3

CASE 3

A 45-year-old male presents with acute collapse and loss of consciousness. He undergoes CT imaging of the brain.

What does the unenhanced CT image (Fig. 7.4) show?

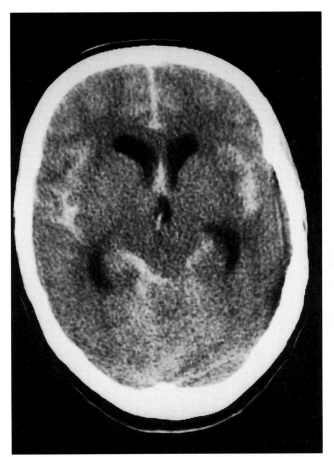

Fig. 7.4

The axial CT image (Fig. 7.4) identifies material of higher attenuation than the brain (looking white on the image) in the subarachnoid space. Normal sulci are not visible; this is an indication of cerebral and cerebellar swelling. The appearances are those of subarachnoid haemorrhage.

Causes of subarachnoid haemorrhage

• Cerebral artery and aneurysmal rupture (the posterior communicating artery within the circle of Willis is the most common site of symptomatic aneurysms).
• Trauma.
• Rare causes include: tumour or infection related subarachnoid haemorrhage, coagulopathy, eclampsia, hypertension.

Figure 7.5 is a further axial CT image of the same patient but at a lower (more caudal) level. The rounded soft tissue mass (arrow) related to the right side of the circle of Willis is an aneurysm arising from the right posterior communicating artery. There is extensive haemorrhage seen in the basal cisterns (curved arrows). This is the cause of the patient's sudden collapse and loss of consciousness.

CT imaging features of subarachnoid haemorrhage

• Focal or widespread blood extending into sulci and outlining gyri.
• Intraventricular blood with the creation of fluid/fluid levels within dependent areas.
• Secondary hydrocephalus as a result of blood in the region of the arachnoid granulations interfering with reabsorption of cerebrospinal fluid.

Further reading

Taber, K.H., Hayman, L.A. & Diaz-Marchan, P.J. (1998) Intracranial haemorrhage. In: *Neuroimaging* (ed. W.W. Orrison, Jr), pp. 863–864. W.B. Saunders Co., Philadelphia.

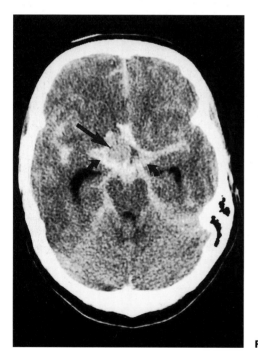

Fig. 7.5

CASE 4

A young patient presents with a rapidly deteriorating level of consciousness after head trauma.

What does this unenhanced CT image (Fig. 7.6) at the skull vertex show?

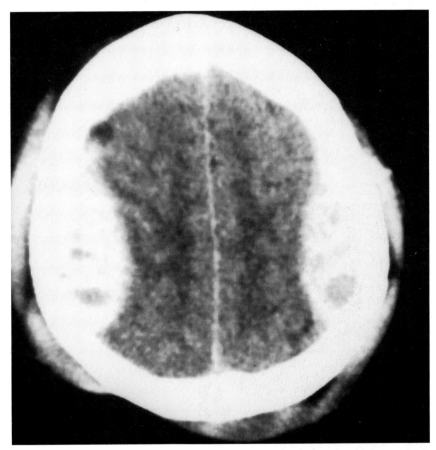

Fig. 7.6

The CT image (Fig. 7.6) reveals bilateral bicon-vex areas of mixed soft tissue and higher-attenu-ation material situated peripherally between the cerebral hemispheres and the parietal bones. There is overlying bilateral scalp swelling. The appearances are those of bilateral extradural haematomas.

Indications for CT imaging following head injury

• Skull fracture with global/focal neurological deficit or seizures.
• Persistent or deteriorating neurological func-tion (i.e. poor or worsening conscious level).

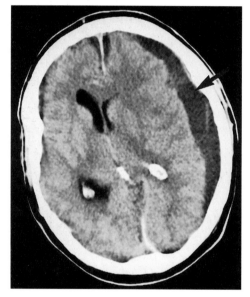

Fig. 7.7

• Depressed skull fracture.
• Penetrating/open skull fracture of vault or base causing cerebrospinal fluid leak.

Features of intracranial, extracerebral haemorrhage on CT imaging

Blood in the brain or meningeal spaces has char-acteristic appearances on CT imaging, which change with the age of the haemorrhage. Within the first 7–10 days the blood is higher density than the brain and appears white. By 3 weeks the blood is isodense with the brain. Beyond this the blood becomes hypodense, appearing black.
1 CT appearance of extradural haemorrhage.
  • Biconvex (lentiform) shape which does not cross suture lines.
  • Cerebral swelling common.
2 CT appearance of subdural haemorrhage.
  • Concavo-convex shape conforming to sub-dural space.
  • Ipsilateral cerebral swelling.
  • Shift of mid-line structures away from con-tained blood with or without obstruction of drainage of the opposite lateral ventricle.

The CT image (Fig. 7.7) illustrates the con-cavo-convex shape formed by a left-sided, chronic subdural haematoma (arrow). There is mid-line shift and the right lateral ventricle is dilated.

Further reading

Taber, K.H., Hayman, L.A. & Diaz-Marchan, P.J. (1998) Intracranial haemorrhage. In: *Neuro-imaging* (ed. W.W. Orrison, Jr), pp. 863–864. W.B. Saunders Co., Philadelphia.

CASE 5

A radiograph (Fig. 7.8) from a barium enema examination in a patient with diarrhoea and abdominal pain is shown.

What changes are seen within in the large bowel?
What abnormal features are seen in the region of the liver?

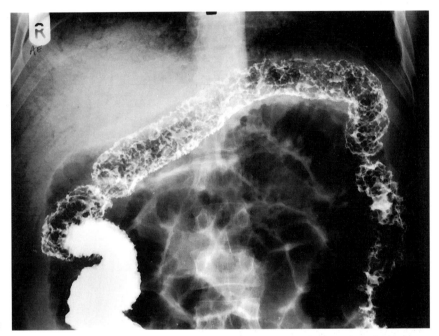

Fig. 7.8

The barium enema radiograph (Fig. 7.8) shows ulceration throughout the colon, giving a cobblestone appearance to the mucosa. Many of the ulcers are too deep to be limited to the mucosa alone, indicating involvement of the submucosal region. The appearance is typical of Crohn's colitis.

Throughout the periphery of the liver there is a branching pattern of fine lucent lines. This represents gas in the portal veins. Gas in the biliary tree has a more central distribution.

Causes of portal venous gas

• Bowel necrosis.
• Inflammatory bowel disease (spontaneous or induced during barium enema/colonoscopy).
• Blunt abdominal trauma.

• Iatrogenic, e.g. endoscopic sphincterotomy or umbilical vein catheterization.
• Peptic ulceration or small bowel obstruction.
• Small bowel obstruction.

Gas in the portal vein is usually regarded as a sign of major intra-abdominal pathology with frequently a fatal outcome. However, it may be iatrogenic, as it was in this case, provoked by air insufflation during the barium enema examination. The radiological features were transitory and the patient asymptomatic!

Further reading

Hong, J.J., Gadaleta, D., Rossi, P., Esquivel J. & Davis, J.M. (1997) Portal vein gas, a changing clinical entity. *Archives of Surgery* **132**, 1071–1075.

CASE 6

A 73-year-old woman presents with a 3-day history of constipation and severe, colicky abdominal pain.

What does the supine abdominal radiograph (Fig. 7.9) show?

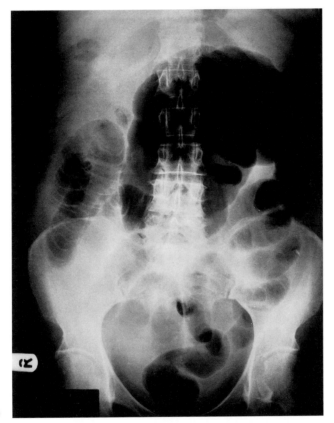

Fig. 7.9

The abdominal radiograph (Fig. 7.9) demonstrates small bowel dilatation together with marked distension of a centrally positioned loop of large bowel. The features are those of intestinal obstruction.

When interpreting radiographs showing intestinal obstruction, it is helpful to establish whether the caecum is in a normal position. In this case, the caecum cannot be seen in the right iliac fossa and this should immediately raise the suspicion of a caecal volvulus with secondary small bowel dilatation as a result of back-pressure through an incompetent ileocaecal valve.

Caecal volvulus

- Abnormally mobile caecum sharing its mesentery with the terminal ileum.
- Rotation usually clockwise with shift towards the mid-line or left hypochondrium.
- Accounts for 2% of intestinal obstruction in adults (less common than sigmoid volvulus).

- May arise secondary to a more distal obstructing colonic lesion e.g. carcinoma.
- Not infrequently a late complication of laparotomy or gynaecological procedures.
- Significant mortality rate (20%), particularly if associated with mesenteric vascular torsion.

Barium enema will confirm the diagnosis and was performed in this case. Figure 7.10 shows centrally positioned caecum and a smooth tapering at its junction with the ascending colon (arrow): a characteristic appearance of caecal volvulus. No obstructing lesion distal to the volvulus was apparent.

Further reading

Szucs, R.A., Wolf, E.L., Gramm, H.F. *et al.* (2000) Miscellaneous abnormalities of the colon. In: *Textbook of Gastrointestinal Radiology* (eds R.M. Gore & M.S. Levine), 2nd edn, pp. 1089–1122. W.B. Saunders Co., Philadelphia.

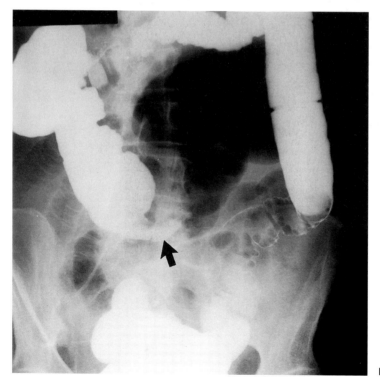

Fig. 7.10

CASE 7

A 71-year-old patient presents with acute onset of bloody diarrhoea and abdominal pain.

Describe the abnormal features on the supine abdominal radiograph (Fig. 7.11).
What is the diagnosis and how may this be confirmed?

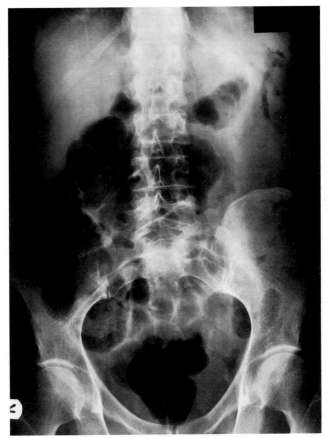

Fig. 7.11

The abdominal radiograph (Fig. 7.11) shows a scalloped outline to the gas in the descending and proximal sigmoid colon, described as 'thumbprinting', with a normal appearance of the more proximal large bowel. The areas of bowel involved are narrowed. The appearances are those of ischaemic colitis. This is confirmed on barium enema examination (Fig. 7.12) with 'thumbprinting' (arrows) due to mucosal oedema, spasm of the affected segment and mucosal ulceration. Interestingly, a delayed study may reveal complete resolution, smooth stricture formation or continued mucosal ulceration.

Ischaemic colitis occurs as a result of decreased perfusion. As in this case, the most commonly affected segments are those of the distal transverse and descending colon. This area reflects a 'watershed' between the vascular supply of the middle colic and inferior mesenteric arteries.

Risk factors for the development of ischaemic colitis

- Obstruction of the large bowel (20% of cases).
- Cardiovascular disease (arrhythmias, emboli, thrombosis).
- Hypovolaemic states.
- Radiation.
- Polycythaemia rubra vera.
- Trauma.

Further reading

Szucs, R.A., Wolf, E.L., Gramm, H.F. *et al.* (2000) Miscellaneous abnormalities of the colon. In: *Textbook of Gastrointestinal Radiology* (eds R.M. Gore & M.S. Levine), 2nd edn, pp. 1089–1122. W.B. Saunders Co., Philadelphia.

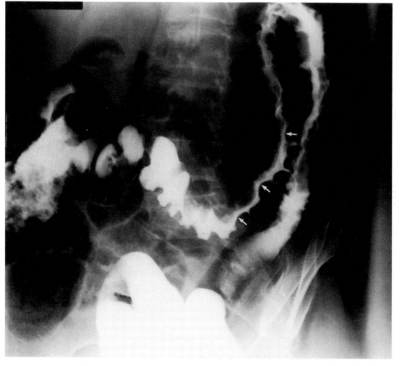

Fig. 7.12

CHAPTER 7

CASE 8

This 68-year-old patient complains of a chronic headache and noticeable swelling of the scalp.

What does this lateral skull radiograph (Fig. 7.13) show?
What is the likely diagnosis?

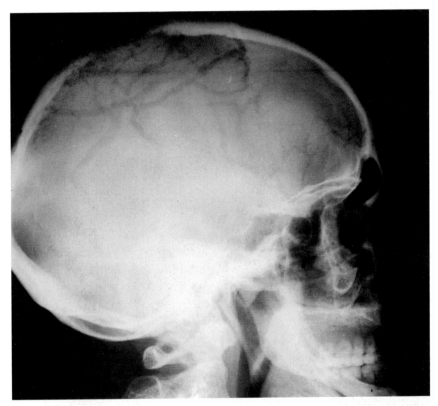

Fig. 7.13

The lateral skull radiograph (Fig. 7.13) reveals a poorly defined destructive lucent area in the vertex of the skull vault together with enlargement of the adjacent vascular channels. This appearance is indicative of an underlying meningioma.

Meningioma

• Attached to dura mater.
• Most common sites include the convexity, parasagittal (falcine), the spheroid ridge and prontobasal.
• Usually benign.
• Indolent growth pattern.
• Symptoms and signs depend upon location.
  The diagnosis is usually reached on CT or MR imaging where meningiomas generally appear well defined and enhance avidly following contrast administration. Some associated oedema/ gliosis is common. Additionally, meningioma may be associated with hyperostosis or calcification, best demonstrated with CT.

A postcontrast coronal CT image (Fig. 7.14) of the same patient shows a large parasagittal mass of high attenuation (large arrow), enhancing vessels in the interhemispherical fissure (small arrows), erosion of bone and extension of the tumour through the skull vault into the scalp. There is oedema/gliosis in the left parietal lobe (open arrow) with compression of the left lateral ventricle.

Further reading

Goldberg, H.I., Lavi, E., & Atlas, S.W. (1996) Extra-axial brain tumours. In: *Magnetic Resonance Imaging of the Brain and Spine* (ed. S.W. Atlas), 2nd edn, pp. 424–446. Lippincott-Raven, Philadelphia.

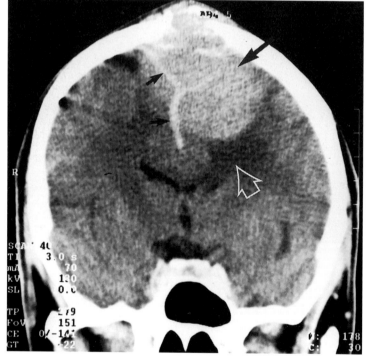

Fig. 7.14

CHAPTER 7

CASE 9

A 34-year-old woman presents with recent-onset, intermittent pelvic discomfort. There is no history of menstrual irregularity.

What are the findings on this radiograph (Fig. 7.15) of the pelvis?
What does the arrow (Fig. 7.15) highlight?
What is the diagnosis?

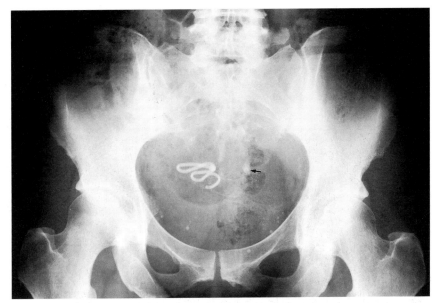

Fig. 7.15

The pelvic radiograph (Fig. 7.15) reveals an intrauterine contraceptive device (IUCD) displaced to the right. Within the left hemipelvis there is a rounded, lucent area which is separate from the gas and faeces in the rectum. There is an area of calcification (arrow) overlying the left lateral margin of the sacrum. These appearances are suggestive of a dermoid cyst of the ovary.

Dermoid cysts (benign teratoma) of the ovary

• Derived from multipotential embryonal germ cells retained within the ovary.
• Usually unilateral.
• Hair, teeth, bone, fat and sebaceous material are often present.

The presence of a well-defined lucent mass of fat density within the pelvis of a female is characteristic of a dermoid cyst. The presence of a tooth, calcification or bone is diagonstic. A firm diagnosis can be reached in 40% of cases on radiograph alone. Ultrasound of the pelvis will further strengthen diagnostic confidence when features of a well-defined, complex cyst containing echogenic material and acoustic shadowing from calcium, bone or tooth are demonstrated. CT or MR imaging may also be used to reveal the characteristic features already mentioned.

CT image (Fig. 7.16) of the same patient shows the predominantly fatty density mass (arrow) in the left side of the pelvis with calcification in its medial wall (curved arrow). It is pushing the rectum to the right. The IUCD is seen in the body of the uterus (open arrow) anterior to the rectum.

Further reading

Hall, D.A. & Hann, L.E. (1993) Gynecologic radiology: benign disorders. In: *Radiology, Diagnosis—Imaging—Intervention* (eds J.M. Taveras & J.T. Ferrucci), Vol. 4, pp. 4–5. J.B. Lippincott Co., Philadelphia.

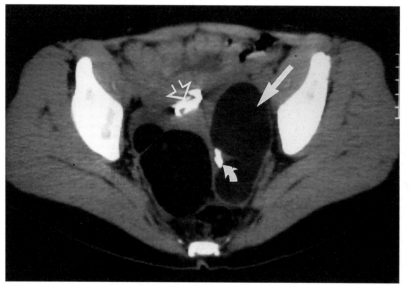

Fig. 7.16

CASE 10

A 43-year-old male presents with epigastric discomfort, early satiety and intermittent, though copious, vomiting. A barium meal was performed.

What key features are evident on this oblique radiograph (Fig. 7.17) of the stomach and duodenum?
List the differential diagnoses.

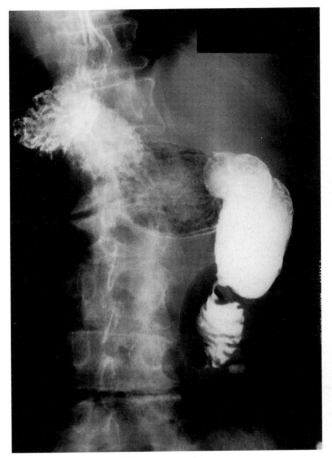

Fig. 7.17

The barium meal radiograph (Fig. 7.17) demonstrates a tight stricture of the second part of the duodenum. Its margins are smooth with no evidence of ulceration. There is marked dilatation of the duodenum proximal to the stricture.

Causes of duodenal obstruction in adults

• Pancreatic: annular pancreas, acute pancreatitis, pseudocyst formation, tumour.
• Duodenal: chronic ulceration, tumour, embryological duplication intramural haematoma.
• Extrinsic compression/involvement: lymph node enlargement, aneurysm, congenital bands, renal tumour.

This patient's clinicoradiological features were the result of an annular pancreas. A wide range of imaging modalities is used, either alone or in conjunction to reach this diagnosis. Endoscopic retrograde cholangiopancreatography (ERCP) is an invasive method of demonstrating the pancreatic duct anatomy, with endoscopic ultrasound and magnetic resonance cholangiopancreatography (MRCP) representing non-invasive alternatives. The presence of oral contrast medium at the site of narrowing is necessary to gain good resolution using CT imaging. This is not always successful and the only abnormality detected may be enlargement of the pancreatic head.

Annular pancreas

• A rare, congenital malformation of the pancreas.
• Failure of normal development and rotation of the ventral buds result in partial or complete encircling of the duodenum by pancreatic tissue.
• Almost 50% of cases present in adult life.
• Association with other anomalies such as malrotation or Down's syndrome may draw attention to its presence in the neonatal period or childhood.
• Pancreatitis or peptic ulceration is a recognized complication.

Further reading

Shirkhoda, A., Gore, R.M. & Ghahremani, M.D. (2000) Anomalies and anatomic variants of the pancreas. In: *Textbook of Gastrointestinal Radiology* (eds R.M. Gore & M.S. Levine), 2nd edn, pp. 1754–1766. W.B. Saunders Co., Philadelphia.

CASE 11

A young patient with Down's syndrome presents with loss of sensation and weakness in the arms together with spasticity.

Sagittal T1-weighted (Fig. 7.18) and T2-weighted (Fig. 7.19) MR images were performed of the cervical and thoracic spine.

What structure is highlighted (open arrow) on the T2-weighted image (Fig. 7.19)?

What abnormality, highlighted by the small arrows, is present on both images?

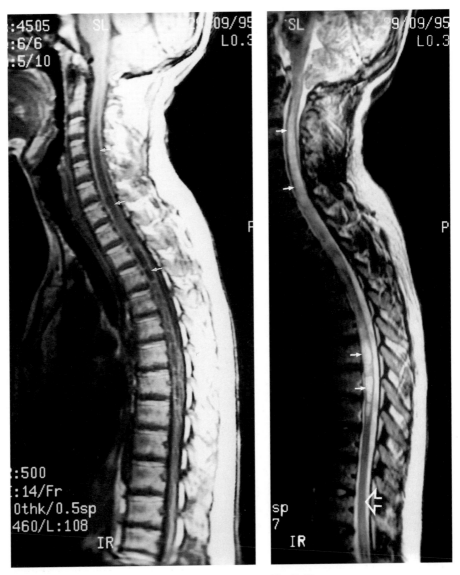

Fig. 7.18   **Fig. 7.19**

The structure highlighted (open arrow) on the T2-weighted image (Fig. 7.19) is the spinal cord. The higher-signal cerebrospinal fluid (CSF) is seen to surround the cord at this level.

The abnormality seen on both sequences (Figs 7.18 & 7.19) is a lobulated cavity extending from C2 to T8 within the substance of the spinal cord. Its signal is isodense with CSF. This is a case of syringohydromyelia.

Syringomyelia is the presence of a fluid-filled cavity, isointense with CSF, extending over several segments within the spinal cord. The cavity lies outside the central canal of the spinal cord. Hydromyelia is the condition of dilatation of the central spinal cord. The two cannot be distinguished on imaging and therefore these abnormalities are described radiologically as syringohydromyelia.

Causes of syringohydromyelia

Congenital
Chiari malformations: associated with other congenital abnormalities, e.g. Klippel–Feil and other vertebral anomalies, meningomyelocele and Down's syndrome.

Acquired
• Post-traumatic (observed in 60% of patients who present with new symptoms after spinal cord injury).
• Arachnoid scarring (post-meningitis, post surgery).
• Post-radiotherapy.

Once the syrinx has been identified, close inspection of the posterior fossa and upper cervical region should be performed. A sagittal T1-weighted MR image (Fig. 7.20) of the brain in this patient shows herniation of the cerebellar peduncles through the foramen magnum to lie in the upper cervical region (arrow). The fourth ventricle is normally positioned (curved arrow). This is a Chiari I malformation.

Further reading

Trowit, C.L. & Barkovich, A.J. (1996) Disorders of brain development. In: *Magnetic Resonance Imaging of the Brain and Spine* (ed. S.W. Atlas), 2nd edn, pp. 183–188. Lippincott-Raven, Philadelphia.

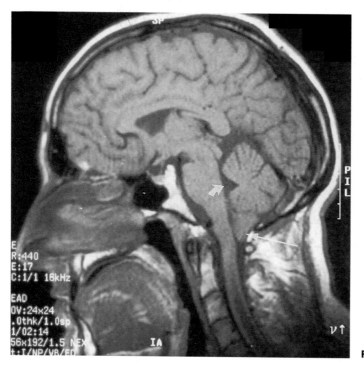

Fig. 7.20

CASE 12

An elderly male patient presented with increasing constipation and urinary outflow difficulties. Digital rectal examination revealed a grossly enlarged prostate compressing the rectum. Rigid sigmoidoscopy confirmed this feature and a normal mucosal appearance was noted.

What abnormality is shown on the barium enema radiograph (Fig. 7.21)? What is the differential diagnosis?

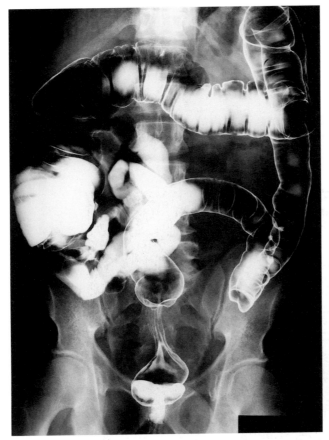

Fig. 7.21

The barium enema radiograph (Fig. 7.21) shows a smooth, tapered narrowing of a short segment of the rectum with no evidence of mucosal ulceration. These are the appearances of extrinsic compression of the rectum.

Differential diagnosis of extrinsic compression of the rectum

- Pelvic neoplasia (e.g. benign and malignant prostate, uterus, ovary).
- Pelvic lymphadenopathy.
- Haematoma/abscess formation.
- Rare causes including endometriosis, amyloidosis and pelvic lipomatosis.

The CT image (Fig. 7.22) confirms circumferential narrowing of the rectum by prostatic tissue (arrow). This was a case of benign prostatic hypertrophy.

Key barium enema features that point towards the cause of luminal narrowing

- Intraluminal: usually cause a roughly hemispherical filling defect which has an acute angle of contact with the wall of the bowel.
- Intramural: smooth or ulcerated mucosa which when malignant is often associated with shouldering, giving an 'apple-core' appearance.
- Extrinsic: smooth narrowing with no mucosal abnormality unless the extrinsic pathology has resulted in direct mucosal involvement.

Further reading

Szucs, R.A., Wolf, E.L., Gramm, H.F. *et al.* (2000) Miscellaneous abnormalities of the colon. In: *Textbook of Gastrointestinal Radiology* (eds R.M. Gore & M.S. Levine), 2nd edn, pp. 1089–1122. W.B. Saunders Co., Philadelphia.

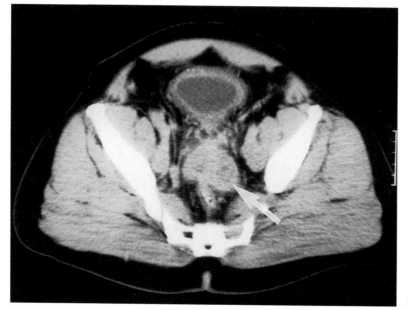

Fig. 7.22

CHAPTER 7

CHAPTER 8

David F. Sallomi

CASE 1

This 76-year-old male presented with abdominal pain and back pain. Examination revealed an expansile abdominal mass.

Postcontrast CT imaging was performed and images at the level of the renal arteries (Fig. 8.1) and more caudally (Fig. 8.2) are included.

What abnormalities are demonstrated?
What is the structure highlighted? (Fig. 8.2, arrow)?
What is the diagnosis?

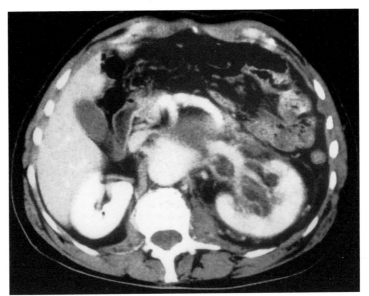

Fig. 8.1

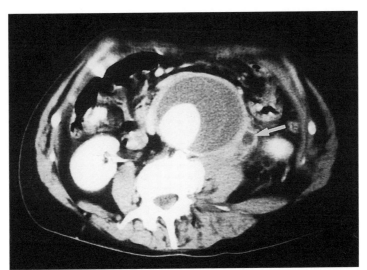

Fig. 8.2

Contrast-enhanced CT images (Figs 8.1 & 8.2) demonstrate a 9-cm maximum diameter abdominal aortic aneurysm with a patent central lumen. The wall of the aneurysm is thickened and irregular and there is associated, adjacent, soft tissue attenuation stranding, especially posterolaterally to the left. This merges with the left psoas muscle and encircles the left ureter which is dilated and obstructed (Fig. 8.2, arrow).

The proximal extent of the aneurysm is above the renal arteries (Fig. 8.1). Note the pelvicalyceal dilatation of the left kidney due to an obstructed left ureter. The term 'perianeurysmal retroperitoneal fibrosis' has been used to describe ureteric obstruction that has resulted from fibrosis around an abdominal aortic aneurysm. The aneurysm is often referred to as 'inflammatory'.

Inflammatory aortic aneurysm

• Accounts for 15% of all abdominal aneurysms.
• The inflammatory infiltrate has similar histological features to idiopathic retroperitoneal fibrosis.
• Ureteric involvement is evident in up to 23% of patients.
• Associated with an elevated erythrocyte sedimentation rate.
• Disease progress responds to corticosteroids.

Although ultrasound examination may demonstrate the thickened wall of an inflammatory aortic aneurysm and accurately assess its maximum diameter, CT imaging is the modality of choice for diagnosis.

Key features of an inflammatory aortic aneurysm on CT imaging

• Thickened aortic wall which may be thinner posteriorly and posterolaterally. These are likely areas of rupture.
• There is a dense desmoplastic reaction within the periaortic tissues that leads to increased attenuation within the retroperitoneal and periaortic soft tissues.
• Desmoplastic reaction can involve the duodenum, inferior vena cava, left renal vein and ureters.

Further reading

Rayder, S.M. (1995) Infected aortic aneurysm. Case report and imaging evaluation. *Clinical Imaging* **19**, 20–24.

CASE 2

This 82-year-old female patient presents with severe epigastric and chest pain with vomiting of acute onset.

What does the erect chest radiograph (Fig. 8.3) show?
What is the diagnosis?
What further investigation is indicated?

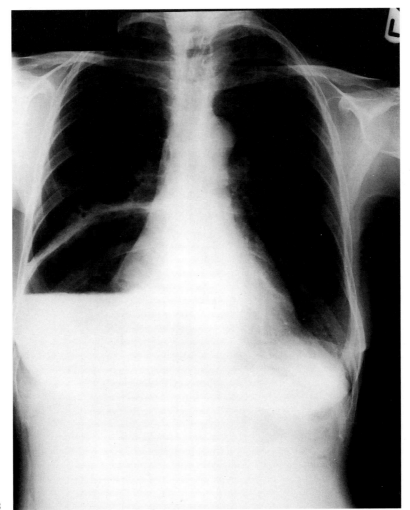

Fig. 8.3

The erect chest radiograph (Fig. 8.3) demonstrates a large air-filled viscus within the right lower zone. It has a thickened, ill-defined superior margin. Bronchovascular markings can be seen through this air-filled viscus. These features suggest an intrathoracic viscus rather than elevation of the right hemidiaphragm. Note the absence of the gastric air bubble under the left hemidiaphragm. These features are consistent with an intrathoracic volvulus of the stomach.

The barium meal examination (Fig. 8.4) confirms a dilated and intrathoracic stomach with an abrupt obstruction to outflow. A nasogastric tube has been advanced into the body of the stomach (arrow). The presence of a gastric volvulus was confirmed at surgery.

Gastric volvulus is due to an abnormal degree of rotation of the stomach (greater than 180°) and takes two principal forms:

• *organo-axial*: rotation around a line extending from the cardia to the pylorus; and

• *mesentero-axial*: rotation around an axis from the lesser curve to the greater curve of the stomach.

Key clinical features of gastric volvulus

• Pain, ineffective vomiting and failure to pass nasogastric tube.
• Initially few abdominal signs.
• Difficult to distinguish clinically from myocardial infarction.
• An abdominal radiograph can be diagnostic: massively distended stomach in the left upper quadrant extending into the chest with paucity of distal bowel gas.

Further reading

Wasselle, J.A. & Norman, J. (1993) Acute gastric volvulus: pathogenesis, diagnosis, and treatment. *American Journal of Gastroenterology* **88**, 1780–1784.

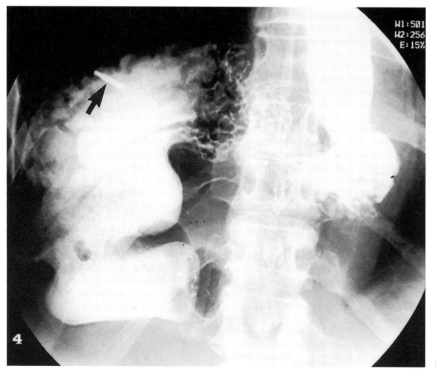

Fig. 8.4

CASE 3

This 48-year-old female with a past history of breast cancer presents with abdominal pain and progressive constipation. No abdominal or pelvic masses were palpable and rigid sigmoidoscopy revealed normal rectal mucosa.

What is the main finding on this oblique view of the sigmoid colon from a barium enema (Fig. 8.5) series?

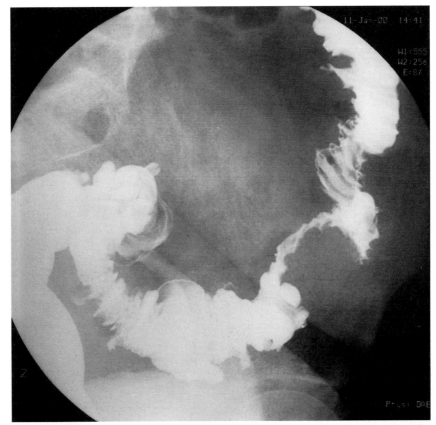

Fig. 8.5

This barium enema radiograph (Fig. 8.5) demonstrates a lobular extrinsic filling defect involving the sigmoid colon, producing significant narrowing of the lumen. The mucosa overlying this eccentric mass has an irregular outline reflecting fine ulceration and implying local infiltration of the colonic wall. Note is made also of diverticular changes within the sigmoid colon.

Causes of extrinsic colonic compression

• Inflammatory mass/abscess, e.g. diverticular disease.
• Metastatic carcinoma.
• Endometriosis.
• Miscellaneous: distended bladder, benign ovarian mass, mesenteric cyst.

Subsequent contrast-enhanced CT imaging (Fig. 8.6) demonstrates an abnormal soft tissue attenuation mass within the left iliac fossa (large arrow). There is a small air bubble within it (small arrow). The abnormal sigmoid loop has thickened walls with irregular soft tissue stranding extending into the pericolic fat and the mesentery. There is also evidence of free fluid within the left iliac fossa.

Histology of the mass revealed metastatic breast cancer.

Colonic involvement by metastatic cancer

• Transcoelomic spread, e.g. ovarian cancer with widespread peritoneal seeding, particularly into the pouch of Douglas.
• Direct, e.g. gastric and pancreatic cancer may extend along transverse mesentery.
• Haematogenous/lymphatic, e.g. breast cancer and malignant melanoma.

Further reading

Forstner, R., Chen, M. & Hricak, H. (1995) Imaging of ovarian cancer. *Journal of Magnetic Resonance Imaging* **5**, 606–613.

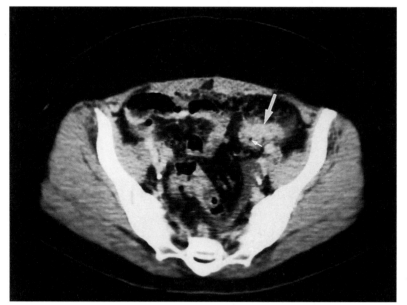

Fig. 8.6

CASE 4

This 45-year-old intravenous drug abuser presents with pain and tenderness within the right groin, fever and right leg swelling.

What features are observed on this radiograph (Fig. 8.7) of the upper right femur?
What is the underlying abnormality?

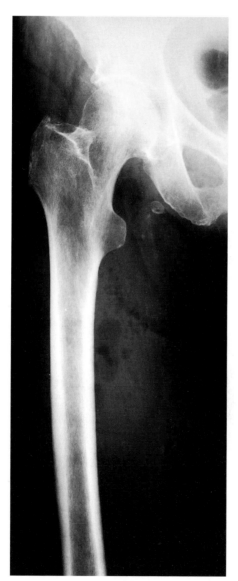

Fig. 8.7

CHAPTER 8   **191**

This radiograph of the right femur (Fig. 8.7) demonstrates multiple lucent areas of varying sizes within the oedematous soft tissues of the thigh and groin. These radiological features are classic for a soft tissue abscess due to gas-forming organisms.

Contrast-enhanced CT imaging (Fig. 8.8) confirms a 4-cm ovoid mass of low attenuation, consistent with an abscess, within the groin (arrow) with multiple bubbles of gas within it (small arrows). Massive oedema within the musculature and subcutaneous tissue of the right thigh is clearly evident when compared with the left.

Complications of intravenous drug abuse

1 Cardiovascular:
  • endocarditis,
  • embolism,
  • pseudoaneurysm formation and arteriovenous fistula.
2 Musculoskeletal:
  • osteomyelitis and septic arthritis,
  • soft tissue infections.
3 Pulmonary:
  • septic emboli.
4 Gastrointestinal:
  • necrotizing enterocolitis and liver abscess.
5 Genitourinary:
  • focal or segmental glomerulosclerosis secondary to immune complex deposition.
6 Neurological:
  • spinal and epidural abscess,
  • meningitis and cerebral abscess.
7 Transmission of infectious disease:
  • hepatitis,
  • HIV.

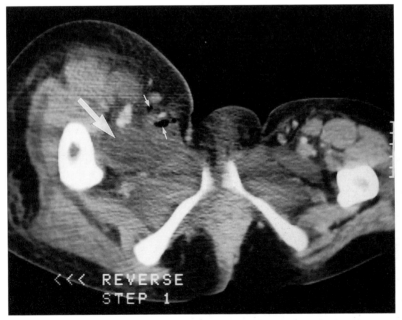

Fig. 8.8

CASE 5

This young patient was involved in a head-on vehicle collision and presents with severe back pain.

What abnormalities are present on this anteroposterior (AP) radiograph view of the lumbar spine (Fig. 8.9)?

What further radiographic view would you request?

What is the underlying diagnosis?

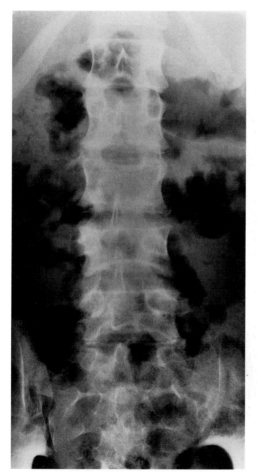

Fig. 8.9

The AP radiograph (Fig. 8.9) demonstrates the hallmark widening of the interspinous distance at the L3 level. The spinous process appears lower in position and is slightly displaced to the right. This appearance is described as 'the empty hole sign', denoting the unusual feature of the L3 vertebral body. The pedicles of the L3 are not well defined.

Trauma must always be evaluated with radiographs in two orthogonal plains. A lateral radiograph (Fig. 8.10) is mandatory. This demonstrates the horizontal fracture extending through the vertebral body, neural arch and spinal process. Note the widening of the posterior part of the intervertebral disc space of L3 and L4, together with the separation of the posterior elements reflecting the flexion injury (arrows). This is a Chance or seat-belt fracture.

Chance fracture

- Seat-belt restraining injury.
- Distraction force applied in flexion.
- Most occur at L2 or L3.
- Associated with retroperitoneal and abdominal visceral injuries.

Further reading

Vollmer, D.G. & Gegg, C. (1997) Classification and acute management of thoracolumbar fractures. *Neurosurgery Clinics of North America* **8**, 499–507.

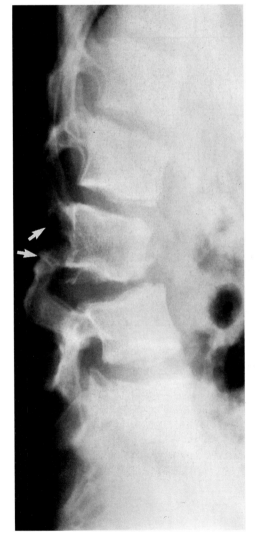

Fig. 8.10

CASE 6

This Asian patient presents with a long history of foot skin infection with multiple sinus formation.

What do the radiographs (Fig. 8.11) of the right foot show?
What is the pathological process?
What is the underlying diagnosis?

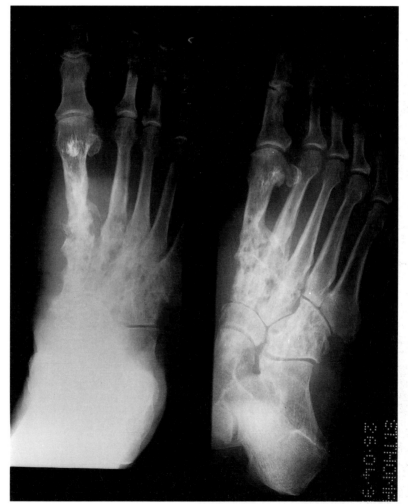

Fig. 8.11

There is widespread ill-defined bony destruction with sclerosis and periosteal new bone formation centred around the tarsometatarsal joints (Fig. 8.11). Extensive soft tissue swelling is also evident. The radiographic changes are those of chronic osteomyelitis.

In this instance the cause is streptomyces infection; the condition is commonly referred to as 'Madura foot'. This disease is seen primarily in the tropics with only rare cases occuring in temperate areas. Countries with the highest reported cases include Sudan, India and Senegal.

Madura foot

- Chronic fungal infection.
- The infective agents are primarily saprophytic micro-organisms found in soil and on plant matter.
- Predisposing factors include trauma, agricultural work, poor personal hygiene, poor nutrition and the presence of wounds.
- The foot is most commonly affected (70%).
- Initially limited to the skin and subcutaneous tissue but may spread through fascial planes to underlying muscle and bone.
- Blood or lymphatic dissemination is unusual.

MR imaging provides a sensitive indicator of bone marrow involvement and therewith disease activity in osteomyelitis. Figure 8.12 is an axial T1-weighted postcontrast-enhanced MR image of the same patient's foot. In addition to the severe bony destruction there is widespread abnormal enhancement within the marrow of the tarsal/metatarsal bones and surrounding soft tissue (see arrows).

Further reading

Venugopal, P.V. & Venugopal, T.V. (1990) Actinomadura madurae mycetomas. *Australasian Journal of Dermatology* **31**, 33–36.

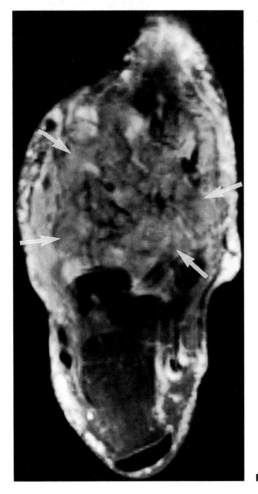

Fig. 8.12

CASE 7

This neonate presents with vomiting and absolute constipation.

What diagnostic features are present on this barium enema radiograph (Fig. 8.13)?

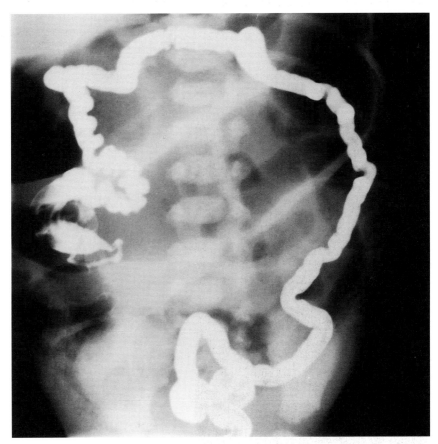

Fig. 8.13

The barium enema radiograph (Fig. 8.13) demonstrates an abnormal, small-calibre colon with several small filling defects within the caecum and terminal ileum. These represent plugs of meconium. Multiple dilated small bowel loops are conspicuous.

Features of 'microcolon' secondary to meconium ileus are evident—this patient has cystic fibrosis.

Meconium ileus

- Neonatal intestinal obstruction.
- Bile-stained vomitus and abdominal distension.
- Palpable distended loops of bowel.
- Some 75–80% due to cystic fibrosis.
- Water-soluble contrast enema may achieve both diagnosis and treatment.
- Volvulus, perforation and atresia are complications.

Plain radiograph features of meconium ileus

- Ground-glass or speckled 'soap-bubble' appearance due to meconium and air is seen within the right upper/lower quadrants (Neuhauser's sign).
- Multiple dilated small loops with paucity of air/fluid levels.
- Microcolon (the colon is underdeveloped).
- Prenatal perforation may lead to chemical peritonitis with adhesions and calcification of the peritoneum, bowel and scrotum.

Further reading

McAlister, W.H. & Kronemer, K.A. (1996) Emergency gastrointestinal radiology of the newborn. *Radiologic Clinics of North America* **34**, 819–844.

CASE 8

This premature 2-day-old baby presents with bloody diarrhoea and systemic upset.

What are the plain abdominal radiograph (Fig. 8.14) findings?
What is the underlying diagnosis?

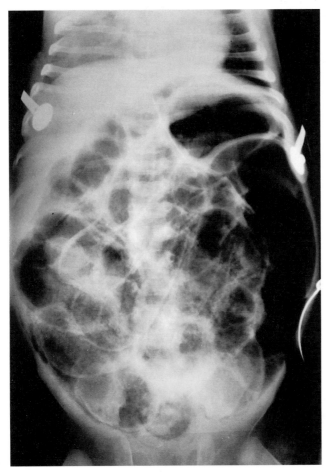

Fig. 8.14

The plain abdominal radiograph (Fig. 8.15 reproduced from Fig. 8.14) demonstrates a speckled appearance to the pathologically dilated bowel with intramural gas adopting rounded and longitudinal configurations (large arrows). A pneumoperitoneum outlines both sides of the bowel wall (Rigler's sign). On closer inspection air is seen within the portal veins (small black arrows).

The diagnosis is necrotizing enterocolitis. All the key radiological features are demonstrated. Barium enema is contraindicated. Complications include stricture formation and bowel perforation.

Necrotizing enterocolitis

• Eighty per cent of cases arise in premature infants.

• Outbreaks can occur in mini-epidemics.
• The causative organism has yet to be isolated.
• Acute inflammation occurs, with mucosal ulceration and widespread transmural necrosis.
• In full-term infants it may be associated with Hirschsprung's disease and other causes of bowel obstruction (atresia, pyloric stenosis, meconium ileus).

Further reading

Buonomo, C. (1999) The radiology of necrotizing enterocolitis. *Radiologic Clinics of North America* **37**, 1187–1198.

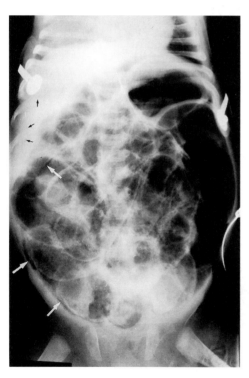

Fig. 8.15

CASE 9

This newborn presents with persistent vomiting and secondary dehydration.

What diagnosis can be reached after study of this anteroposterior (AP) radiograph (Fig. 8.16)?

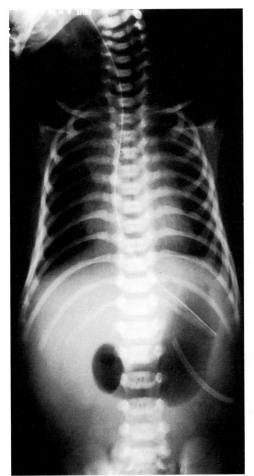

Fig. 8.16

This plain radiograph (Fig. 8.16) demonstrates a nasogastric tube with a gastrostomy feeding tube. The stomach and duodenal cap are air-filled with an absence of more distal bowel gas secondary to duodenal obstruction.

Neonatal duodenal obstruction may be the result of atresia, stenosis, duodenal web, intra-luminal diverticulum, duodenal duplication cyst, annular pancreas, or peritoneal (Ladd) bands secondary to incomplete intestinal rotation. In this instance the diagnosis is duodenal atresia.

Duodenal atresia

• Congenital duodenal obstruction.
• Abnormality is caused by defective vacuoliza-tion of the duodenum between weeks 6 and 11 of fetal life.
• Eighty per cent occur distal to the ampulla of Vater.
• Down's syndrome is associated in 30% of cases.

• May have associated anomalies (VATER syndrome).

Key plain radiographic features seen in duodenal atresia

• 'Double bubble sign'—gas/fluid levels in the duodenal bulb and gastric fundus.
• Absence of gas within the remainder of the small and large bowel.
• Any colon that is visualized is of normal calibre.

Further reading

Dalla Vecchia, L.K., Grosfeld, J.L., West, K.W., Rescorla, F.J., Scherer, L.R. & Engum, S.A. (1998) Intestinal atresia and stenosis: a 25-year experience with 277 cases. *Archives of Surgery* **133**, 490–496; discussion 496–497.

CASE 10

This 58-year-old female has a known history of carcinoma of the cervix and previous radical radiotherapy. She has complained of bloody diarrhoea and intermittent lower abdominal pain.

What does the lateral view (Fig. 8.17) from the barium enema examination show?
Suggest the underlying diagnosis.

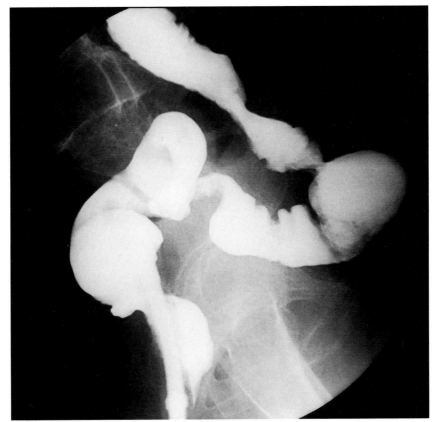

Fig. 8.17

The barium enema radiograph (Fig. 8.17) demonstrates stricture formation in the rectum and sigmoid colon. Although the overlying mucosa is irregular in outline there is no evidence of shouldering. Radiation-induced stricture formation is most probable. This is supported by subsequent CT imaging (Fig. 8.18). The abnormal rectum has enhanced irregular thickened walls (arrows) and increased attenuation within the perirectal fat, creating a 'halo effect'.

Chronic radiation enteritis may present months to years after the completion of therapy or it may begin as acute enteritis and persist after the cessation of treatment. Between 5% and 15% of patients treated with radiation develop chronic problems. Treatment for carcinoma of the cervix is commonly implicated.

Barium enema features of radiation enteritis

• Serrated bowel margin with thickened folds and ulceration.
• Multiple strictures which may cause partial bowel obstruction.
• Wall thickening and separation of bowel loops. Shortening of affected small bowel.
• Fistula formation.

Further reading

Donner, C.S. Pathophysiology and therapy of chronic radiation-induced injury to the colon. *Digestive Diseases* **16**, 253–261.

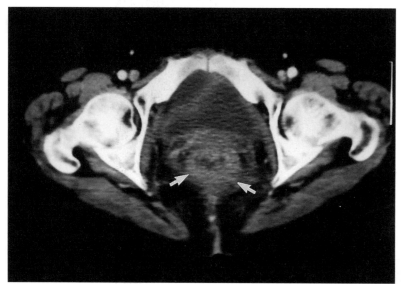

Fig. 8.18

CASE 11

This 78-year-old patient presents with vomiting, absolute constipation and fever.

What are the main radiographic features seen in this supine abdominal radiograph (Fig. 8.19)?

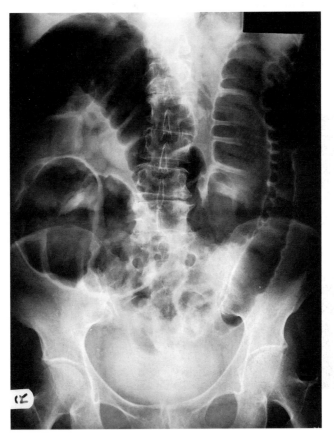

Fig. 8.19

The supine abdominal radiograph shows evidence of distal large bowel obstruction with pneumoperitoneum (Fig. 8.19).

The underlying cause was an obstructing carcinoma of the distal sigmoid colon which had perforated.

Radiographic features

Radiographic features of pneumoperitoneum on the supine abdominal radiograph include:
- *Rigler's sign.* Air on both sides of the wall of the colon thereby defining, equally well, both the outer wall of the colon and the surface of the lumen. A magnified view of the caecal area (Fig. 8.20) demonstrates this phenomenon. The caecal wall is delineated by air (arrows).

- *Football sign.* Large pneumoperitoneum producing a large central lucency to the abdomen.
- *Doge's cap sign.* Triangular collection of gas in Rutherford Morison's pouch.
- *Telltale triangle sign.* Triangular pocket of air between three loops of bowel.
- *Inverted V sign.* Outlining both lateral umbilical ligaments.

Further reading

Williams, N. & Everson, N.W. (1997) Radiological confirmation of intraperitoneal free gas. *Annals of the Royal College of Surgeons of England* **79**, 8–12.

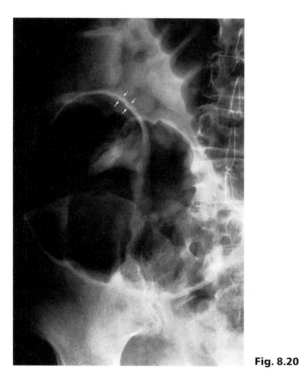

Fig. 8.20

CASE 12

This 6-month-old infant presents with vomiting and passage of bloody/mucous stools.

What does the supine abdominal radiograph (Fig. 8.21) show?
What is the diagnosis?

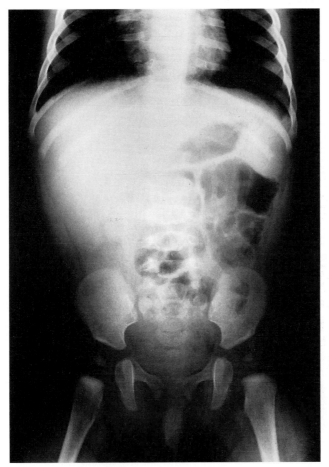

Fig. 8.21

The plain radiograph (Fig. 8.21) demonstrates several air-filled small bowel loops, a paucity of bowel gas within the right iliac fossa and a soft tissue mass within the epigastrium. A crescent of gas outlines the intussuscepted bowel.

A radiograph (Fig. 8.22) from the barium enema series demonstrates a lobular filling defect as a result of intussuscepted bowel (arrows). The caecum is pulled up by the intussusception and lies in the right upper quadrant. An image later in the series (Fig. 8.23) confirms reduction of the intussusception with barium refluxing into the small bowel (curved arrows).

Aetiology of childhood intussusception

1 Idiopathic (95% of cases) presumably related to lymphoid hyperplasia and mesenteric adenitis.
2 Lead point (5% of cases), e.g.
  • Meckel's diverticulum;
  • enteric polyp or mass;
  • Henoch–Schönlein purpura;
  • inspissated meconium.

Radiological treatment in children with intussusception

• Air or water reduction using ultrasound guidance.
• Barium reduction with confirmation of free flow into the ileum (Fig. 8.23).
• Recurrence rate of 10% within 48 hours.
• Contraindicated in patients with obvious acute abdomen (signs of peritonitis or perforation).

Further reading

Del-Pozo, G., Albillos, J.C., Tejedor, D. *et al.* (1999) Intussusception in children: current concepts in diagnosis and enema reduction. *Radiographics* **19**, 299–319.

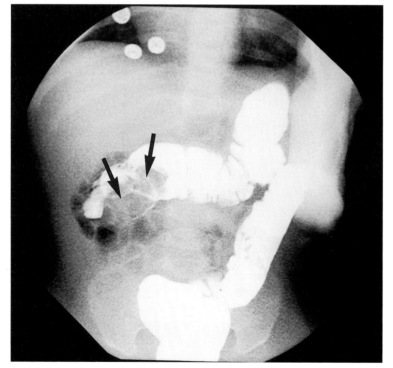

Fig. 8.22

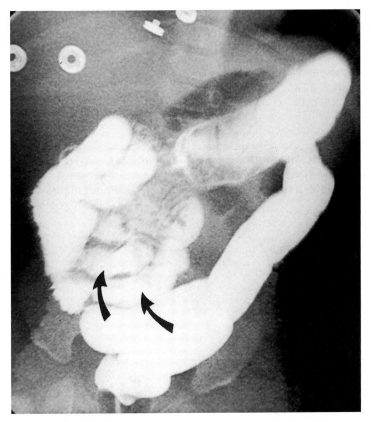

Fig. 8.23 Barium enema reduction of intussusception confirmed by the presence of contrast refluxing into small bowel (curved arrows). Compare with preceding figures.

GLOSSARY

Orientation of radiological images

Presentation of all radiological images, unless otherwise stated, follows a conventional format throughout the chapters of this book. Radiographs have been obtained in anteroposterior, lateral or oblique projection. Ultrasound images are orientated such that the body surface lies superiorly. Computed tomography (CT) or magnetic resonance (MR) images are viewed caudiocranially. The ventral and dorsal surfaces are positioned, respectively, superiorly and inferiorly. Images configured as a sagittal or coronal section will be identified in the text.

Ultrasound imaging

Ultrasound is a high-frequency mechanical vibration produced by a transducer constructed of a piezoelectric material. These ultrasonic waves travel through tissues by the transfer of energy from particle to particle. As the wave crosses a boundary between two tissues, of differing acoustic impedance, a reflection is produced which is detected by the probe and relayed as an image on the screen. The non-reflected waves are unavailable to imaging. Conversely, where reflection is total and all the energy is returned, an acoustic shadow is created. Bone, calcification or air produces this effect and the more distal tissues cannot be visualized.

The signal intensity observed on the ultrasound screen is referred to as echogenicity. The brighter the reflected signal (e.g. from a calculus), the higher the echogenicity and the more likely to cast an acoustic shadow. Fluid is seen as a hypoechoic area (very dark on the screen). Loss of the signal in fluids paradoxically creates a brighter image beyond, referred to as acoustic enhancement.

Computed tomography imaging

This technique utilizes the rotation of an X-ray beam using numerous detectors, enabling a computer-created composition of cross-sectional images or 'slices'. This information can be accrued more rapidly by moving the patient through the rotating X-ray beam (spiral CT imaging). This obtains a continuous spiral volume of tissue and enables three-dimensional reconstructions and angiographic imaging.

The extent to which tissues absorb the X-rays is referred to as attenuation. The greater the level of absorption, the higher the attenuation and the whiter the image. Conversely, low attenuating tissue is dark. The quantity of absorption, with reference to that obtained with water, is measured in Hounsfield units (HU).

Tissue	Hounsfield units (HU)
Air	−400 to −600
Fat	−60 to −100
Water	*0*
Soft tissues	+40 to +80
Bone	+400 to +1000

Negative values represent low attenuation and positive values represent high attenuation.

Improved resolution of tissue can be gained by combining the administration of iodinated contrast orally/rectally or intravenously while simultaneously accruing the radiological images. Contrast enhancement of the tissues is achieved. Intravenous iodinated contrast enhancement may be either vascular or parenchymal (extravascular). Abnormal tissue is highlighted as it will have different enhancement characteristics to those of the parent organ.

Magnetic resonance imaging

Radiofrequency radiation, not X-rays, in combination with high-intensity magnetic fields is utilized in this technique. Predominantly, the hydrogen nucleus and its characteristics in association with water and lipid are mapped out. Different tissues reflect characteristic signals and the contrast resolution of soft tissue is superior to that obtained by CT imaging. Computer reconstruction can likewise obtain three-dimensional images. Moreover, intravenous contrast using a gadolinium chelate can be utilized for enhancement.

Two basic parameters are utilized for MR imaging analysis: longitudinal relaxation time (T1) and transverse relaxation time (T2). Tissues can be characterized by these parameters; liquids have long T1 and T2 relaxation times whereas those of soft tissues are much shorter. Solids are characterized by a long T1 and short T2 time.

By varying the radiofrequency and/or magnetic field gradient, different features can be highlighted in tissues, thereby exposing pathological processes. These changes of parameters are termed sequences.

Sequence	Tissue characteristics
T1-weighted	Fat has a high signal intensity whereas fluid has a low signal intensity. Soft tissues are intermediate. Good anatomical tissue definition is gained
T2-weighted	Fat has a lower signal intensity whereas fluid has a high signal intensity. Soft tissues are intermediate. Oedema (increase in extracellular and interstitial fluid) will return a high signal
Contrast enhancement using intravenous gadolinium chelate	Causes a local paramagnetic effect. The contrast agent leads to a high signal on T1-weighted images

Contraindications to MR imaging include the presence of the following ferromagnetic materials that may move, or become displaced, in the magnetic field:
- intracranial aneurysm clips and haemostatic vascular clips;
- prosthetic heart valves;
- otological and ocular implants;
- electrical devices including pacemakers;
- some intravascular coils, stents and filters.

INDEX

ureteric transitional cell carcinoma
  91–2
urethral stricture 90
urinary frequency 83
urinary outflow obstruction 181
urinary tract infection
  emphysematous pyelonephritis
    153–4
  in infants 89–90
  tuberculosis 83–4

vaginal discharge 103–4
valvulae conniventes 62
vestibular schwannoma 57–8

volvulus
  caecal 169–70
  gastric 187–8
  and gastric outlet obstruction 160
  of sigmoid colon 41–2
vomiting 51, 143, 145, 159, 177, 197, 205

Warthin's tumour 78
water-lily sign 122
weight loss 21, 91, 93, 101, 155
widened teardrop sign 32
wrist, carpal instability 95–6

Yersinia enterocolitica 464